I0702087

Atkins Diet for Beginners

Embark on a transformative journey of weight loss. Unlock the potency of low-calorie living, cultivating a lasting, healthy lifestyle. enriched with 110 delicious recipes.

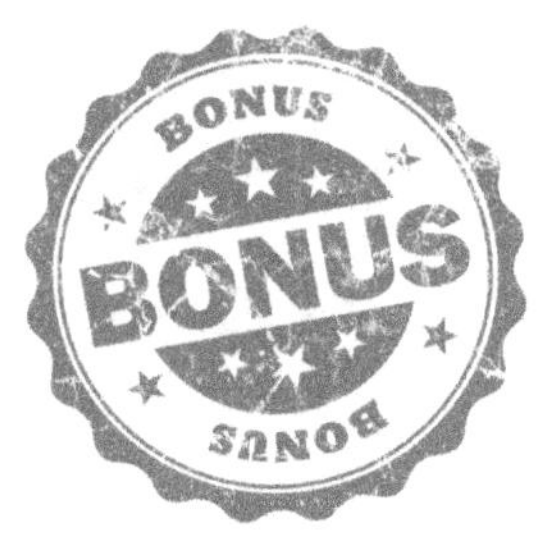

30-DAYS LOW-CARB MEAL PLAN

Thelma J. Curtis

Copyright © 2023 Thelma J. Curtis

All rights reserved. No part of this book may be reproduced, distributed, or transmitted in any form or by any means, including photocopying, recording, or other electronic or mechanical methods, without the prior written permission of the author, except in the case of brief quotations embodied in critical reviews and certain other noncommercial uses permitted by copyright law.

This book is provided for informational purposes only and is not intended as a substitute for professional medical advice, diagnosis, or treatment. The author and publisher make no representations or warranties regarding the accuracy or completeness of the information provided. Individuals using the information in this book do so at their own risk.

Before making any significant changes to your diet or lifestyle, it is advisable to consult with a qualified healthcare professional or nutritionist. The author and publisher disclaim any responsibility for adverse effects or consequences resulting directly or indirectly from the use of the information in this book.

Any references to specific products, brands, or services are for informational purposes only and do not constitute an endorsement or recommendation by the author or publisher.

While every effort has been made to ensure the accuracy and completeness of the information presented, the author and publisher assume no responsibility for errors or omissions or for damages resulting from the use of the information contained herein.

<u>Bonus:30-Days Low-Carb Meal Plan</u>

Week 1

Day 1:
- Breakfast: Avocado and Bacon Breakfast Wrap
- Lunch: Greek Chicken Salad
- Dinner: Mushroom and Spinach Stuffed Chicken
- Snack: Keto Cheesecake Bites

Day 2:
- Breakfast: Keto Blueberry Muffins
- Lunch: Zucchini and Chicken Enchiladas
- Dinner: Salmon and Avocado Lettuce Wraps
- Snack: Caprese Egg Bake

Day 3:
- Breakfast: Coconut Flour Porridge with Almonds
- Lunch: Turkey and Bacon Lettuce Cups
- Dinner: Cauliflower Fried Rice with Chicken
- Snack: Almond Butter and Celery Sticks

Day 4:
- Breakfast: Spinach and Feta Breakfast Muffins
- Lunch: Tuna Salad Stuffed Bell Peppers
- Dinner: Shrimp and Zucchini Noodles
- Snack: Avocado Tuna Boats

Day 5:
- Breakfast: Keto Pancakes with Sugar-Free Syrup
- Lunch: Caprese Zoodle Salad
- Dinner: Turkey and Avocado Lettuce Wrap

- Snack: Cottage Cheese and Berry Bowl

Day 6:
- Breakfast: Baked Avocado Eggs
- Lunch: Pesto Chicken Salad Lettuce Wraps
- Dinner: Eggplant Lasagna
- Snack: Grilled Lemon Garlic Chicken

Day 7:
- Breakfast: Greek Yogurt Breakfast Bowl
- Lunch: Beef and Broccoli Stir-Fry
- Dinner: Cobb Salad with Ranch Dressing
- Snack: Turkey and Vegetable Stir-Fry

Week 2:

Day 8:
- Breakfast: Low-Carb Yogurt Parfait
- Lunch: Chicken and Broccoli Alfredo Bake
- Dinner: Turkey and Avocado Lettuce Wrap
- Snack: Chocolate Avocado Mousse

Day 9:
- Breakfast: Greek Yogurt with Berries and Nuts
- Lunch: Spinach and Feta Stuffed Bell Peppers
- Dinner: Lemon Dill Baked Cod
- Snack: Buffalo Cauliflower Bites

Day 10:
- Breakfast: Keto Pancakes with Sugar-Free Syrup
- Lunch: Pesto Zoodle Bowl with Grilled Chicken
- Dinner: Asparagus and Ham Stuffed Chicken
- Snack: Avocado and Bacon Deviled Eggs

Day 11:
- Breakfast: Almond Flour Waffles
- Lunch: Tuna Salad Stuffed Bell Peppers

- Dinner: Cajun Shrimp and Sausage Skillet
- Snack: Cucumber and Cream Cheese Bites

Day 12:
- Breakfast: Cottage Cheese and Berry Bowl
- Lunch: Eggplant Parmesan
- Dinner: Caprese Zoodle Salad
- Snack: Parmesan Crisps

Day 13:
- Breakfast: Turkey and Avocado Lettuce Wrap
- Lunch: Creamy Mushroom and Spinach Scramble
- Dinner: Chicken Alfredo with Spaghetti Squash
- Snack: Hard-Boiled Eggs with Dill

Day 14:
- Breakfast: Keto Blueberry Muffins
- Lunch: Grilled Chicken Caesar Salad
- Dinner: Turkey and Vegetable Stir-Fry
- Snack: Chocolate Almond Butter Delight

Week 3:

Day 15:
- Breakfast: Avocado Tuna Boats
- Lunch: Creamy Avocado and Shrimp Salad
- Dinner: Brussels Sprouts and Bacon Skillet
- Snack: Lemon Coconut Bliss Balls

Day 16:
- Breakfast: Zucchini and Cheese Fritters
- Lunch: Egg Salad Cucumber Boats
- Dinner: Turkey and Bacon Lettuce Cups
- Snack: Spicy Guacamole with Jicama Sticks

Day 17:

- Breakfast: Caprese Egg Bake
- Lunch: Cajun Shrimp and Sausage Skillet
- Dinner: Broccoli Cheddar Stuffed Chicken Breast
- Snack: Parmesan Crisps

Day 18:
- Breakfast: Keto Pancakes with Sugar-Free Syrup
- Lunch: Turkey and Avocado Lettuce Wrap
- Dinner: Spaghetti Squash Carbonara
- Snack: Almond Butter and Celery Sticks

Day 19:
- Breakfast: Spinach and Feta Breakfast Muffins
- Lunch: Caprese Zoodle Salad
- Dinner: Lemon Dill Baked Cod
- Snack: Buffalo Cauliflower Bites

Day 20:
- Breakfast: Greek Yogurt Breakfast Bowl
- Lunch: Chicken and Broccoli Alfredo Bake
- Dinner: Turkey and Vegetable Stir-Fry
- Snack: Chocolate Almond Butter Delight

Day 21:
- Breakfast: Keto Blueberry Muffins
- Lunch: Pesto Zoodle Bowl with Grilled Chicken
- Dinner: Salmon and Broccoli Foil Packets
- Snack: Avocado and Bacon Deviled Eggs

Week 4:

Day 22:
- Breakfast: Egg and Avocado Breakfast Bowl
- Lunch: Mediterranean Quinoa Salad
- Dinner: Eggplant Lasagna Roll-Ups

- Snack: Cucumber and Cream Cheese Bites

Day 23:
- Breakfast: Bacon and Spinach Omelette
- Lunch: Spaghetti Squash with Meatballs
- Dinner: Greek Lamb Chops with Tzatziki
- Snack: Parmesan Crisps

Day 24:
- Breakfast: Sausage and Cheese Breakfast Casserole
- Lunch: Asparagus and Feta Stuffed Turkey Burgers
- Dinner: Cauliflower Shepherd's Pie
- Snack: Avocado and Bacon Deviled Eggs

Day 25:
- Breakfast: Mushroom and Feta Frittata
- Lunch: Turkey and Avocado Lettuce Wrap
- Dinner: Zucchini Noodles with Pesto Shrimp
- Snack: Lemon Coconut Bliss Balls

Day 26:
- Breakfast: Keto Pancakes with Sugar-Free Syrup
- Lunch: Caprese Zoodle Salad
- Dinner: Stuffed Bell Peppers with Ground Turkey
- Snack: Spicy Guacamole with Jicama Sticks

Day 27:
- Breakfast: Low-Carb Yogurt Parfait
- Lunch: Egg Salad Cucumber Boats
- Dinner: Cauliflower Crust Pizza
- Snack: Almond Butter and Celery Sticks

Day 28:
- Breakfast: Greek Yogurt with Berries and Nuts
- Lunch: Grilled Chicken Caesar Salad
- Dinner: Creamy Garlic Parmesan Chicken

- Snack: Avocado and Bacon Deviled Eggs

Day 29:
- Breakfast: Avocado Tuna Boats
- Lunch: Creamy Avocado and Shrimp Salad
- Dinner: Turkey and Vegetable Stir-Fry
- Snack: Chocolate Almond Butter Delight

Day 30:
- Breakfast: Low-Carb Yogurt Parfait
- Lunch: Eggplant Lasagna Roll-Ups
- Dinner: Grilled Lemon Garlic Chicken
- Snack: Lemon Coconut Bliss Balls

Week 5-8:
Continue rotating through the Week 1-4 recipes and introduce some new recipes.

Note:
- Adjust portion sizes based on individual nutritional needs.
- Ensure to stay hydrated with water throughout the day.
- Customize the plan to meet your dietary preferences and requirements.

This meal plan offers variety, flavor, and nutrition while adhering to the principles of the Atkins diet.

About the Thelma J. Curtis

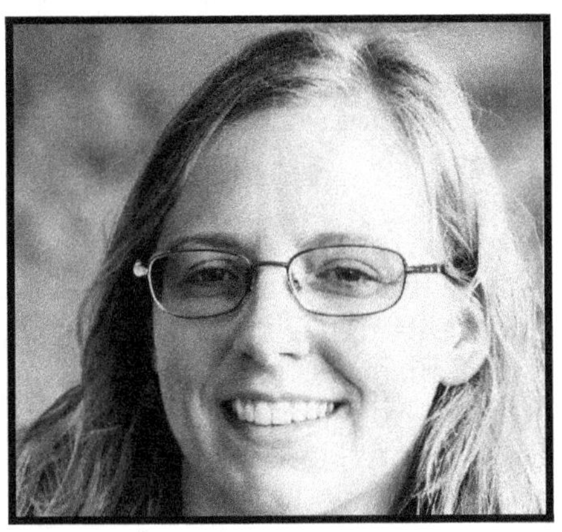

Thelma J. Curtis is a passionate advocate for health and wellness, dedicating her expertise to guide individuals towards a balanced and fulfilling lifestyle. With a background in nutrition and a commitment to helping others achieve their weight loss goals, Thelma has become a trusted voice in the field of holistic well-being.

Thelma's journey in nutrition began with a personal quest for a sustainable and effective weight loss solution. Her exploration led her to discover the transformative power of the Atkins diet. Motivated by her own success and the desire to share this life-changing approach, Thelma embarked on a mission to empower others to achieve optimal health.

As a certified nutritionist and wellness coach, Thelma combines her academic knowledge with a practical understanding of the challenges individuals face in adopting healthier lifestyles. Her writing reflects a compassionate and realistic approach, making complex dietary concepts accessible to beginners and seasoned wellness enthusiasts alike.

In addition to her educational background, Thelma's recipes are a testament to her creativity and passion for flavorful, yet nutritious, meals. Through her book, "Atkins Diet for Beginners 2023," Thelma invites readers to embrace a journey of balanced nutrition, time-tested strategies, and delicious recipes that pave the way to lasting wellness.

Thelma J. Curtis's commitment to promoting a healthier world extends beyond her writing. She continues to engage with her audience through online platforms, providing ongoing support, insights, and inspiration. Join Thelma on this transformative journey, and let her expertise guide you towards a lifestyle of vitality, balance, and sustainable weight loss.

Table of Contents

Introduction

Greetings and welcome to 'Atkins Diet for Beginners,' your starting point for a life-changing path to a more vibrant, healthy version of yourself. This extensive book explores the relationship between diet, time, and weight reduction, revealing the power of a low-calorie lifestyle to develop a long-lasting, healthy way of living. This book, which is enhanced with 110 delectable recipes, is your road map to healthy eating and long-term weight reduction, guaranteeing vigor at every turn. Set off on this inspiring journey to learn the tenets that make Atkins a tried-and-true method for reaching your health objectives.

Why the Atkins diet is effective

The Atkins diet is intended to function by adjusting the body's metabolism by consuming less carbohydrates. Reducing the amount of carbs consumed causes the body to go into ketosis. During ketosis, the body burns stored fat instead of glucose, or sugar, as its main energy source. This change in metabolism may result in a number of things that may explain why the Atkins diet works so well:

1. Increased Fat Burning: When the body has less glucose available for energy, it burns more fat stored in its fat reserves, which may contribute to weight reduction.

2. Stabilized Blood Sugar Levels: The diet helps control blood sugar levels by limiting the amount of

carbohydrates consumed, which lessens the spikes and crashes brought on by high-carb meals. Better energy management and appetite control may result from this.

3. Enhanced Satiety: The Atkins diet emphasizes the importance of foods high in protein and healthy fats, which tend to be more satiating. This may result in consuming less calories overall, which will help with weight control.

4. Lower Insulin Levels: Insulin levels are typically lower when a diet lower in carbohydrates is consumed. Since insulin is a hormone that encourages fat accumulation, reduced amounts may help people lose weight.

5. Preservation of Lean Muscle Mass: Maintaining overall metabolic health during weight reduction requires lean muscle mass to be preserved, which is made possible by an adequate protein intake in the Atkins diet.

6. Improved Lipid Profile: Research indicates that the Atkins diet may have a beneficial effect on lipid profiles, resulting in higher triglyceride and cholesterol levels.

Recognizing the Interaction of Time, Diet, and Weight Loss

Comprehending the interplay between diet, time, and weight reduction is essential for attaining long-lasting and efficient outcomes in your health quest. The cornerstone is nutrition, which fuels your body's complex functions like gasoline. You may affect your metabolism and energy levels by choosing the right meals to eat at the right times.

Time is an important factor in this calculation, and it includes both the length of your meals and the sustained dedication to a lifestyle. As your body adjusts to new eating patterns, patience becomes an asset, and regular, healthy behaviors eventually provide noticeable benefits.

One of the main objectives of many people is to lose weight, which is a complex result of how time and nutrition interact. Making nutrient-dense, low-calorie meal choices helps maintain a healthy energy balance, and making these decisions consistently over time results in long-term weight control.

The Atkins diet's advantages

There are a number of possible advantages to the Atkins diet, however each person's experience may differ. Here are a few often mentioned benefits:

1. Weight Loss: Losing weight with the Atkins diet is often successful. The diet may lower total calorie intake and enhance fat burning by encouraging the consumption of protein and healthy fats while lowering carbohydrate intake.

2. Appetite Control: Meals high in fat and protein are often more satisfying, making people feel filled for longer. Better appetite control and less snacking may result from this.

3. Better Blood Sugar Levels: The Atkins diet may help control blood sugar levels by reducing the consumption

of high-glycemic carbs. Those who have type 2 diabetes or insulin resistance may benefit most from this.

4. Improved Lipid Profile: Research indicates that the Atkins diet may have a beneficial effect on lipid profiles, resulting in lower triglyceride and cholesterol levels.

5. Preservation of Lean Muscle Mass: The Atkins diet's sufficient protein consumption helps to avoid muscle wasting by maintaining lean muscle mass throughout weight reduction.

6. Enhanced Energy: By switching from burning carbohydrates for energy to burning fat for energy (ketosis), one may avoid the energy crashes and spikes that come with high-carb meals and have more steady energy levels throughout the day.

7. Decreased Cravings: Cutting down on carbohydrates might encourage healthy eating choices by reducing sugar cravings and reliance on processed foods.

8. Emphasis on Whole Foods: Vegetables, lean meats, and healthy fats are highlighted in the Atkins diet, which promotes the intake of whole, unprocessed foods.

9. Beneficial Metabolic Changes: The diet may result in favorable modifications to metabolic indicators, such as inflammatory and insulin-sensitive markers.

10. Modifiable Phases: The Atkins diet is divided into stages that let people alter the plan according to their tastes and objectives. Long-term sustainability is aided by this flexibility.

Chapter 1
Foundations of the Atkins Diet

The Basics of Atkins: Principles and Philosophy

The principles and outlook of the Atkins diet distinguish it from other conventional eating plans. The following are the basic principles of the Atkins diet:

1. Carbohydrate Restriction: The cornerstone of the Atkins diet is the intentional restriction of carbohydrate intake. The diet aims to induce ketosis by reducing carbohydrate intake, particularly from processed grains and simple sugars.

2. Phased Approach: There are two phases to the Atkins diet, each with a different purpose. The first phase, which is also called the Induction Phase, is the most carbohydrate-restricted. Subsequent phases gradually reintroduce more carbohydrates, allowing for a tailored and sustainable approach.

3. Emphasis on Healthy Fats and Protein: The Atkins diet places a strong emphasis on consuming healthy fats and protein while limiting carbohydrates. While meals rich in healthy fats encourage satiety and serve as a replacement energy source, meals high in protein

provide the essential amino acids for preserving muscle mass.

4. Ketosis: Achieving and maintaining a state of ketosis is one of the core principles of the Atkins diet. The state known as ketosis is reached when the body begins to use fat stores as its primary energy source rather than glucose. This process is thought to hasten the decrease of fat.

5. Tailored Approach: The Atkins diet is flexible since it recognizes that different individuals have different goals for weight loss and different carbohydrate tolerances. It enables the adoption of a personalized approach based on an individual's hobbies, way of life, and health.

6. Focus on entire Foods: The diet encourages consuming entire foods that are rich in nutrients, such as vegetables, lean meats, nuts, and seeds. Consume less processed and refined foods.

7. Blood Sugar Management: By cutting down on high-glycemic carbohydrates, one of the objectives of the Atkins diet is to assist with blood sugar regulation. This may be particularly beneficial for those who are searching for blood sugar stability or who have insulin resistance.

8. Long-Term Well-Being: In addition to weight loss, the Atkins diet is marketed as a lifestyle approach that fosters long-term well-being. It also attempts to address overall metabolic health, energy levels, and mental clarity in addition to weight reduction.

What Sets Atkins Apart: A Comparative Overview

The Atkins diet differs from other dieting approaches due to its unique phases and guiding principles. Below is a list of comparisons that illustrate how Atkins differs from a few well-known diets:

1. The Atkins Keto Diet: Allows for a progressive increase in the quantity of carbs taken in.
   - Keto: To maintain ketosis, often follows a low-carb, high-fat diet.

2. The diet known as Paleo: Atkins: Because of its historical roots, this diet places a strong emphasis on cutting carbohydrates without specifically banning any foods.
   Paleo: Emphasizes whole, unprocessed meals that humans would have consumed in the Paleolithic.

3. Mediterranean Diet:
   - Atkins: Reduces the intake of carbohydrates, including those that are often regarded as healthy, such as whole grains and fruits.
   - Mediterranean: A focus on whole grains, fruits, vegetables, and healthy fats is combined with a moderate intake of protein.

4. Low-Calorie Diet:
   - Atkins: Places more emphasis on the macronutrient composition than calorie counting.
   Low-Calorie: emphasizes reducing calories in general rather than macronutrient ratios.

5. Low-Fat Diet:

- Atkins: Promotes the utilization of healthy fats as a primary energy source.
   - Low-Fat: Restricts the amount of fat in eating, often emphasizing carbohydrates and lean proteins.

6. Atkins Intermittent Fasting This may be changed to allow for intermittent fasting, but there are no time limits for the fast.
   - Intermittent Fasting: This mode of eating and fasting alternates between periods.

7. Plant-Based/Vegetarian Diet:
   - Atkins: This diet allows the use of animal products, in contrast to an exclusively plant-based diet.
   - Plant-Based: Stresses meals made mostly of plants and steers clear of or uses animal products sparingly.

8. Dietary Strategies to Lower Blood Pressure, or DASH Diet:
   - Atkins: Allows for a larger fat intake; may differ in terms of fat and carbohydrate consumption.
   - DASH: Prioritize fruits, vegetables, lean meats, and low-fat dairy products to help decrease blood pressure.

Chapter 2
Nutrition Unveiled

The Role of Nutrition in Weight Loss

The quantity, composition, and effects on the body of the calories consumed by an individual are greatly influenced by their diet. Important aspects of nutrition's role in weight reduction include the following:

1. Caloric Balance: The primary method of weight loss involves generating a caloric deficit, or an environment in which more calories are burned than are taken in. Nutrition is important because it supplies the necessary fuel and keeps the body in an equilibrium that promotes fat loss.

2. Macronutrient Composition: The body's energy use is influenced by the distribution of proteins, fats, and carbs in the diet. The aim of diets that manipulate macronutrient ratios, such as the Atkins diet, is to optimize fat burning for energy production by the body.

3. Protein for Satiety: Eating enough protein increases feelings of fullness and satiety, which reduces the amount of calories consumed overall. When decreasing weight, it's also crucial for preserving lean muscle mass.

4. Carbohydrate Quality: The kind and quality of carbohydrates are affected. Long-lasting energy is provided by whole, complex carb diets, and reducing the intake of processed sugars reduces blood sugar spikes and cravings.

5. Healthy Fats for Satiety: Eating foods rich in healthy fats, like avocados, almonds, and olive oil, makes individuals feel fuller and makes it easier for them to control how much they eat at a time to avoid overindulging.

6. Micronutrient Density: Consuming a diet rich in nutrients ensures that the body receives the essential vitamins and minerals for optimal function. This is crucial to avoid vitamin deficiencies during weight loss.

7. Meal Timing and Frequency: These factors have an impact on metabolism and appetite. Methods like intermittent fasting focus on adjusting the time of meals to change how the body processes food.

8. Hydration: Staying properly hydrated is crucial for overall health and may aid in weight loss by boosting metabolic processes and preventing the mistaken belief that thirst equals' hunger.

9. Individual Variation: It's important to realize that each individual responds to different eating tactics in a unique way. Numerous variables, like as metabolism rate, lifestyle, and genetics, might affect how the body responds to certain dietary approaches.

10. Durability: Long-term weight loss success often depends on how durable dietary choices are. Finding a diet that suits each person's preferences and can be adhered to regularly over time is the key.

Nutritional Strategies for Long-Term Health

For long-lasting wellness, eating habits that support overall health and well-being must be adopted. Important dietary strategies to promote long-term well-being include the following:

1. Balanced Diet: Eat a balanced diet consisting of macronutrients (fats, proteins, and carbs) to meet your energy needs and support several bodily functions.

2. All Foods Stress: Make whole, highly nutritious, less processed meals a top focus. Lean meats, fruits, vegetables, whole grains, and healthy fats are all beneficial to overall health.

3. Hydration: Ensure that you drink enough amount of water each day. Staying properly hydrated is essential for several physiological processes as well as for overall wellness.

4. Mindful Eating: Pay attention to your body's cues of hunger and fullness while you eat. Try not to get sidetracked during meals and savor the flavors and textures of your food.

5. Color and Variety: Make sure a variety of brightly colored fruits and vegetables are a part of your diet. Different hues often suggest a broad range of components and antioxidants that are health-promoting.

6. Portion Control: Be mindful of portion sizes to avoid overindulging. Using smaller plates and being aware of

your body's signals of hunger and fullness may help with portion control.

7. Lessen Your Consumption of Processed Foods and Added Sugars: Cut down on the quantity of highly processed foods and sugars that you eat. Select complete, nutrient-dense foods to encourage better overall health and blood sugar control.

8. Prioritize Fiber: - Include high-fiber foods including fruits, vegetables, whole grains, and legumes in your diet. Fiber keeps the digestive system healthy, assists in satiety, and enhances overall well-being.

9. Nutritious Fats: - Incorporate foods rich in healthy fats, such as almonds, avocados, seeds, and olive oil. These lipids are essential for both the brain's health and the body's ability to absorb nutrition.

10. Moderation and Enjoyment: Use a reasonable approach that allows for occasional delights in moderation. A balanced diet is essential for overall health.

11. Regular Meals: Aim for regular, balanced meals to provide you with a steady flow of energy throughout the day. It is best to avoid missing meals in order to maintain stable blood sugar levels.

12. Personalized Approach: - Recognize that each individual has unique nutritional needs. A customized dietary plan should include factors such as age, degree of activity, and health issues.

13. Habits for Life: - Focus more on developing enduring habits than on short-term solutions. Improvements that

are sustainable are more likely to lead to long-term well-being.

Chapter 3
Time-Driven
Transformations

Time-Tested Approaches to Weight Loss

Time-tested weight reduction methods include tactics that have shown to be successful time and time again. These are a few timeless ideas:

A calorie deficit, or an excess of calories expended over calories taken, is the basic component of weight reduction. The concept of balancing energy intake and expenditure is ageless.

It has been shown that adopting well-balanced and healthful eating habits that prioritize whole foods, lean meats, fruits, vegetables, and whole grains will help with weight reduction.

A tried-and-true tactic is incorporating regular exercise into your daily routine. Engaging in physical exercise promotes general health and well-being in addition to helping burn calories.

Controlling portion sizes aids in avoiding overindulgence. The practice of mindful eating—aware of your body's signals of hunger and fullness—has shown to be effective over time.

Maintaining proper hydration promotes general health and may help with weight control. A sense of fullness may also be enhanced by drinking water before to meals.

A traditional strategy involves consuming a balance of fats, proteins, and carbs. Every macronutrient supports physiological processes and encourages fullness.

One well-established method of managing weight is to address behavioral elements of eating, such as emotional eating or mindless nibbling.

Having a network of friends, family, or the community behind you may be a source of inspiration and support while trying to lose weight.

Being present and thoughtful while eating is a key component of mindful eating. This method promotes mindful eating and a closer relationship with food.

The secret to good behavior is consistency. Long-term weight control is facilitated by dietary and lifestyle modifications that are sustainable.

Setting high priority for good sleep is an age-old tactic for maintaining general health, including weight control. Sleep deprivation may throw hormone balance off, which can impact metabolism and hunger.

There are long-term advantages to stress management practices including yoga, meditation, and other relaxation approaches. Stress may affect eating habits and make it more difficult to lose weight.

Establishing reasonable, attainable objectives helps one feel accomplished. Over time, little, incremental adjustments are often more sustainable.

Gradually Developing a Sustainable Way of Life

Making small, doable adjustments that support your beliefs and general well-being is the first step in creating a sustainable lifestyle over time. The following fundamental ideas will assist you in developing a healthy and sustainable lifestyle:

1. Set Achievable, Realistic objectives: Make sure your objectives are reasonable and take into account your existing way of life. Then, progressively work toward them. Radical overhauls are less sustainable than small, regular adjustments.

2. Make complete Foods a Priority: Make complete, nutrient-dense foods a major part of your diet. For a balanced diet, include a range of fruits, vegetables, whole grains, lean meats, and healthy fats.

3. Frequent Physical Activity: Include frequent exercise in your schedule, making sure to choose enjoyable activities. To improve total fitness, combine aerobic, strength, and flexibility training.

4. Develop Mindful Eating Habits: During meals, minimize distractions, enjoy tastes, and pay attention to your body's signals of hunger and fullness. This promotes a more positive connection with eating.

5. Hydration: Drink water all day long to be properly hydrated. Water is necessary for many body processes and promotes general health.

6. Balanced Macronutrients: Make sure your meals include an appropriate ratio of fats, proteins, and carbs.

Every macronutrient is essential to maintaining the operations of your body.

7. Quality Sleep: - Make sure you get quality sleep by keeping a regular sleep routine and setting up a comfortable sleeping space. For both emotional and physical health, getting enough sleep is essential.

8. Stress Management: - Include stress-relieving activities in your daily routine, including deep breathing techniques, meditation, or time spent outside. It's critical to stress management for general health.

9. Establish Healthful Routines Slowly: - Establish new routines gradually to give your body time to adjust. Before implementing more adjustments, concentrate on implementing one or two at a time and making them a regular part of your regimen.

10. Create a Supportive Environment: - Be in the company of friends, family, or like-minded people who support you in your efforts to lead a healthy lifestyle.

11. Savor the Process: - Take pleasure in the trip. Savor the little triumphs and the good changes you come across along the path. Having an optimistic outlook helps with sustainability.

12. Lifelong Learning: - Remain receptive to new information on health, fitness, and diet. To make wise decisions, keep learning about healthy living techniques.

13. Adjust to Changing Circumstances: - Realize that life is dynamic and that you may need to make alterations to your schedule. Recognize and adjust to changing conditions without giving up.

14. Self-Compassion: - Treat yourself with kindness. Recognize that obstacles will always arise, and it's important to face them with compassion for yourself. Take lessons from past mistakes and keep going.

Chapter 4
Low-Calorie Living

Unleashing the Power of Low-Calorie Choices

Using low-calorie options to their full potential is a calculated move that will help with weight control and general well-being. To fully reap the advantages of low-calorie alternatives, keep the following points in mind:

1. Nutrient Density: Choose meals that are low in calories yet high in nutrients. Fruits, vegetables, and lean meats are healthy options that are high in vitamins and minerals.

2. Volume Eating: To enhance volume without substantially raising calorie consumption, choose meals rich in water and fiber. This encourages a contented and full feeling.

3. Smart Snacking: To reduce hunger, include low-calorie snacks in between meals. Snacking on fresh veggies, Greek yogurt, or a handful of berries are healthy choices that don't pack on the calories.

4. Hydration: To keep hydrated, make water and other low-calorie drinks a priority. Occasionally, hungry pangs are really indicators of dehydration.

5. Mindful Portions: - Manage your intake by paying attention to serving sizes. Use smaller dishes and plates

to give the impression of bigger amounts without adding too many calories.

6. Lean Proteins: - Opt for lean protein sources like lentils, fish, chicken breast, or tofu. Eat meals high in protein to feel fuller longer while also providing necessary amino acids.

7. Vegetable Focus: - Make veggies the focal point of your meals. They are rich in fiber and other micronutrients in addition to having little calories.

8. Whole Grains: For more fiber and minerals, choose whole grains rather than processed grains. Whole grains may be a component of a tasty, low-calorie meal and help maintain energy levels.

9. Moderate Inclusion of Good Fats: - Incorporate moderate amounts of nuts, avocados, and olive oil, among other sources of healthy fats. Despite having more calories, they provide vital nutrients and aid with satiety.

10. Calorie Awareness: - Gain knowledge about how many calories items include. Having a clear understanding of the energy content of various meals facilitates decision-making.

11. Meal Planning: - Arrange meals ahead of time to guarantee a calorie-controlled and nutritionally balanced diet. This lessens the possibility of making calorie-dense, impulsive decisions.

12. Flexibility and Variety: To guarantee a varied and pleasurable diet, embrace a range of low-calorie items.

This adaptability keeps things interesting and encourages sticking to a balanced diet.

13. Balanced Approach: - Put more of an emphasis on eating a balanced diet than on severely cutting calories. A comprehensive strategy guarantees that your body gets the nourishment it needs to perform at its best.

Formulating a Diet that Equalizes Calorie Consumption and Taste

Making deliberate meal selections and emphasizing filling, nutrient-dense foods are key to creating a diet that strikes a balance between taste and calorie consumption. The following guidelines will help you create a tasty, but calorie-conscious, meal plan:

1. Accept Whole Foods: - Make whole, unprocessed foods the foundation of your diet. In addition to providing vital nutrients, fresh fruits, vegetables, lean meats, complete grains, and healthy fats provide a range of tastes.

2. Herbs and Spices: In order to improve the taste of your food without consuming more calories, use herbs and spices freely. Try different mixes to create intriguing flavor profiles.

3. Lean Proteins: - opt for sources of lean protein such as beans, fish, chicken, or tofu. These choices add to a sensation of fullness in addition to being flavorful.

4. Colorful Variety: Make sure your meals include a range of vibrant fruits and veggies. In addition to adding

variety to your dish, different hues often suggest various food profiles.

5. Mindful Cooking Methods: - To maintain taste without adding too many calories, try cooking methods like grilling, roasting, or sautéing with little to no oil. These techniques bring out the inherent flavors of the food.

6. meal Control: To control calorie consumption, pay attention to meal sizes. Portion sizes that are smaller let you enjoy the taste without going overboard.

7. Healthy Fats: - Incorporate, but only in moderation, foods high in healthy fats, such as nuts, avocados, and olive oil. These fats increase satiety and give foods a richer, more flavorful texture.

8. Balanced Macronutrients: Make an effort to provide meals that are proportionately high in lipids, proteins, and carbs. This improves the flavor experience overall and boosts overall nutrition.

9. Try Different Flavors: - Take chances while cooking. To make your meals interesting and delightful, try different cuisines, taste combinations, and ingredients.

10. Mindful Eating: To properly enjoy the tastes and sensations of your meal, engage in mindful eating. Enjoy every mouthful and be aware of your body's signals of hunger and fullness.

11. Flavored Hydration: - Use citrus, berry, or herb slices to add natural tastes to water. This gives water a revitalizing twist without adding additional calories.

12. Create Balanced Meals: To guarantee a comprehensive and fulfilling experience, create meals that include a range of dietary categories. A well-balanced combination of tastes and textures makes a meal more pleasurable.

13. Treats in Moderation: - Give yourself the occasional treat in moderation. This keeps your food in balance and keeps you from experiencing emotions of deprivation.

14. Culinary Creativity: - Use your imagination while preparing food. Make cooking a fun and rewarding part of your lifestyle by trying out new recipes and modifying old ones.

Chapter 5
Healthy Lifestyle Foundations

The Importance of a Healthy Lifestyle

A healthy lifestyle includes a variety of behaviors and decisions that support mental, emotional, and physical well-being, making it essential for total wellbeing. The following salient points underscore the significance of leading a healthy lifestyle:

1. Disease Prevention: - A healthy lifestyle that includes regular exercise, a balanced diet, and stress reduction may greatly lower the chance of developing chronic conditions including diabetes, heart disease, and certain types of cancer.

2. Physical Health: - Engaging in regular physical exercise improves flexibility, strengthens bones and muscles, and promotes cardiovascular health in addition to general physical fitness.

3. Weight Management: Reaching and maintaining a healthy weight is made easier by leading a healthy lifestyle that includes frequent exercise and a balanced diet. This is crucial to avoiding health problems associated with obesity.

4. Emotional Wellness: A healthy diet and regular exercise both supports improved mental health. Frequent exercise generates endorphins, which help

people feel less stressed and anxious. A balanced diet also promotes healthy brain development.

5. High-quality sleep is encouraged by healthy lifestyle decisions, such as regular sleep schedules and relaxation techniques. Restorative sleep is necessary for both the body and the mind.

6. Enhanced Mood and Enhanced Energy: - Mood and energy levels are favorably impacted by regular exercise, healthy eating, and enough sleep. These routines support a happier and livelier everyday existence.

7. Stress Reduction: Managing stress levels may be achieved by partaking in stress-relieving activities like physical activity, meditation, or time spent in nature. Long-term stress is detrimental to one's physical and emotional well-being.

8. Social Connections: - Social interaction and solid interpersonal ties are often components of a healthy lifestyle. Social ties improve emotional health and provide a network of support during trying times.

9. Enhanced Productivity: Getting enough sleep, eating a balanced diet, and engaging in physical exercise all improve productivity and cognitive performance. Work and everyday activities are favorably impacted by a healthy lifestyle.

10. Longevity: Studies constantly demonstrate that those who lead healthy lifestyles often live longer. Living a longer and healthier life is a result of making wise decisions about nutrition, exercise, and stress reduction.

11. Disease Management: Maintaining a healthy lifestyle is essential for those with pre-existing medical illnesses in order to manage and lessen the effects of disease. It bolsters the efficacy of pharmaceuticals and medical interventions.

12. Preventive Healthcare: - A healthy lifestyle requires regular examinations, screenings, and preventative treatment. Better results and prompt action are made possible by early diagnosis of health problems.

13. Improved Immune Response: - The immune system is strengthened by a healthy diet, consistent exercise, and enough sleep, which lowers the risk of disease and increases the body's capacity to fight infections.

14. Good Practices for Next Generations: - Living a healthy lifestyle provides a good example for kids and the next generation. A lifetime commitment to wellbeing is facilitated by early establishment of good behaviors.

Combining the Atkins Method with Fitness

Your weight reduction and health journey might be more successful overall if you combine exercise with the Atkins method. A high-protein, low-carb diet combined with frequent exercise may help maintain lean muscle mass, encourage fat reduction, and enhance general health. The following factors should be taken into account when combining exercise with the Atkins diet:

1. Cardiovascular Exercise: To promote calorie burning and enhance heart health, regularly engage in cardiovascular exercise. The Atkins method may be enhanced by exercises like cycling, swimming, running, and brisk walking.

2. Strength Training: To develop and preserve lean muscle mass, use strength training activities. Using weights or resistance bands, resistance exercise tones the body and increases metabolism.

3. Flexibility Exercises: To increase range of motion and lower the chance of injury, include stretches and yoga into your routine. Additionally, these pursuits enhance general wellbeing.

4. Exercise Timing: - Take into account when you should schedule your exercises in respect to your Atkins stages. Focus on low-intensity activities during the early stages, when carbohydrate consumption is more limited. As you advance, you may add in more strenuous exercises.

5. Hydration: - Make sure you drink enough of water, particularly if you're exercising. In addition to promoting general health, adequate hydration may assist in addressing any Atkins diet side effects including constipation.

6. Pre- and Post-exercise Nutrition: - Be mindful of your diet before and after your exercise. Have a light snack with some protein and healthy fats before working out. After that, refuel with a healthy lunch or snack to aid in your recuperation.

7. Pay Attention to Your Body: Pay close attention to how your body reacts to exercise, particularly while using the Atkins diet plan. If you feel fatigued, think about modifying the duration or level of intensity of your exercises.

8. Adjust to stages: - Modify your exercise regimen to meet the various Atkins diet stages. Focus on low-intensity activity in the beginning, and as your consumption of carbohydrates rises, progressively add in higher-intensity activities.

9. Set Realistic Goals: - Make sure your fitness objectives are in line with your overall health goals. Having specific objectives may help you customize your workout regimen, whether it's for weight reduction, muscular growth, or increased endurance.

10. Consistency is Key: - Long-term success depends on maintaining consistency in both food and activity. Create a workout regimen that you can stick with and that goes well with your selected Atkins diet strategy.

11. Consult with Professionals: - To make sure that your fitness plan is in line with your health objectives, especially if you are new to exercising or have particular health problems, consider speaking with fitness experts or healthcare specialists.

Chapter 6
Your Guide to Balanced Nutrition

Crafting Nutrient-Packed Meals

When creating nutrient-dense meals that follow the Atkins diet plan, low-carb, high-protein foods should be combined with a range of nutrient-dense items. The following advice may help you prepare tasty, nutrient-dense meals:

1. Select Lean Proteins: - Include lean protein sources including fish, eggs, tofu, poultry, and lean meats. These meals supply important amino acids in addition to being low in carbs.

2. Incorporate a Range of Vegetables: Arrange a wide variety of non-starchy veggies in your dish. Broccoli, cauliflower, zucchini, peppers, and leafy greens are all great options. They have a lot of fiber, vitamins, and minerals.

3. Healthy Fats in Moderation: - Include foods like avocados, almonds, seeds, and olive oil that are moderately high in healthy fats. These fats provide necessary fatty acids and aid in satiety.

4. Whole Grains in Moderation: Add whole grains in moderation if you're at a period when you can consume more carbs. Brown rice, barley, and quinoa may enhance your meals with fiber, vitamins, and minerals.

5. Investigate Low-Carb Vegetables: - Try substituting lower-carb vegetables, such as zucchini noodles or cauliflower rice, for higher-carb ones to boost nutritional density.

6. Incorporate Vibrant Fruits: - As the Atkins diet progresses, gradually incorporate little servings of vibrant fruits like berries. These provide natural sweetness and antioxidants.

7. Include Dairy or Dairy Alternatives: - Add dairy or dairy substitutes to your diet to get calcium and other important elements. Choose low-carb substitutes like almond milk or Greek yogurt.

8. Herbs and Spices for taste: - In order to improve taste without consuming more calories or carbs, use herbs and spices freely. Add some fresh herbs, ginger, garlic, and other spice mixes to your food to make it taste better.

9. Balance Macronutrients: Make an effort to include proteins, lipids, and carbs in each meal in an appropriate proportion. This well-rounded strategy promotes general nutrition.

10. Create Balanced Meals: To guarantee a thorough nutritional profile, create meals that include a range of food categories. A delicious and nourishing meal is made up of a combination of proteins, vegetables, healthy fats, and, if appropriate, whole grains.

11. Drink Water with Your Meals: To keep hydrated, drink water with your meals. In addition to being

beneficial to general health, enough hydration may heighten feelings of fullness.

12. Mindful Cooking Methods: - Employ cooking methods that maintain the nutritious content of the foods. Nutrient-retaining cooking techniques include roasting, grilling, sautéing, and steaming.

13. Experiment with Plant-Based Proteins: - Include sources of plant-based protein, such as tofu, lentils, and beans, in your meals to spice them up and provide more fiber.

14. Portion limit: - To limit calorie intake, use portion control. Consider portion proportions to prevent overindulging.

Recognizing Atkins' Macronutrients

The Atkins diet emphasizes adjusting the consumption of certain macronutrients—carbohydrates, proteins, and fats—to accomplish weight reduction and better general health. Therefore, it is important to understand macronutrients while following the program. The function of each macronutrient in the Atkins diet is broken out as follows:

1. Carbohydrates Role in Atkins: During the first stages of the Atkins diet, a restriction on carbohydrates is implemented to cause a condition known as ketosis, in which the body begins burning fat for energy. This encourages fat reduction and blood sugar regulation.

Phases: The four stages of the Atkins diet are Induction, Balancing, Pre-Maintenance, and Maintenance. During these phases, the consumption of carbohydrates is progressively increased.

Sources: Avoid high-carb meals and concentrate on low-carb veggies throughout the first stages. Add tiny quantities of fruits, legumes, and whole grains in later periods.

2. Proteins Role in Atkins: As they maintain lean muscle mass during weight reduction, proteins are an essential part of the Atkins diet. Protein has a role in satiety as well.

Phases: The Atkins diet places an emphasis on protein consumption at each stage. When carbs are limited during the Induction period, it is very crucial.

3. Fats Role in Atkins Diet: The Atkins diet emphasizes the consumption of healthy fats to meet a large amount of daily energy requirements. Fats support the body's nutritional needs and aid in satiety.

Phases: The Atkins diet incorporates healthy fats at the start and at every stage. Sources including avocados, almonds, seeds, olive oil, and fatty seafood are highlighted.

Comprehending macronutrients within the framework of the Atkins diet entails adjusting their ratios according to the particular stage you are in. A typical guideline for every step is as follows:

During the induction phase, carbohydrates should be consumed in moderation, mostly from non-starchy vegetables (20–25 grams daily).

Proteins: Focused to support the preservation of muscular mass.

Fats: Healthy fats provide a substantial amount of daily energy.

During the balancing phase, increase the amount of carbohydrates by five grams at a time.
Proteins: They still make up a large portion of meals.
Fats: Contribute significantly to daily energy requirements.

Phases of Pre-Maintenance and Maintenance:
Carbohydrates: Modified in accordance with personal tolerance, with the goal of maintaining weight at a certain level.
 Proteins: Continue to be crucial for good health.
 Fats: Remain an important energy source.

Chapter 7
Sustainable Weight Loss Strategies

Long-Term Success with Atkins

In order to follow the Atkins diet for the long term, one must embrace its tenets as a sustainable way of life, including regular exercise, a balanced approach to general well-being, and good eating habits. The following are important factors to take into account in order to succeed with the Atkins diet in the long run:

1. Smooth Transition between Phases: - Adopt the Atkins diet gradually, letting your body adjust to each stage. The probability of long-term success and adherence is raised by this strategy.

2. Adopt a Well-Balanced Diet: As you go through the stages, concentrate on developing a diet that is both balanced and well-rounded. Include a range of meals high in nutrients, such as lean meats, veggies that aren't starchy, healthy fats, and, if necessary, moderate quantities of carbs.

3. Portion Control: Even while eating low-carb items, use portion control to prevent overindulging. Keeping an eye on serving sizes helps with weight control and general wellness.

4. Frequent Physical exercise: - Make time for frequent physical exercise in your daily schedule. Exercise helps

people lose weight, improves their general health, and works best when combined with the Atkins diet.

5. Remain Hydrated: - Drink water all day long to stay adequately hydrated. In addition to promoting several biological processes, hydration may help control appetite.

6. Track Carb consumption: - Continually track your consumption of carbohydrates according to your own tolerance. Observe the effects that various meals have on your body and make adjustments as necessary.

7. Include entire Foods: - Give your diet a high priority for entire, unprocessed foods. Whole foods support general health by offering vital nutrients.

8. Moderate Intake of Healthy Fats: - Incorporate healthy fats in moderation. Although fats play a significant role in the Atkins diet, it's crucial to find a balance and refrain from consuming too much of them.

9. Mindful Eating: Become aware of your hunger and fullness signals while you eat. Being present while eating promotes a more positive connection with food.

10. Regular Check-Ups: Make an appointment with a healthcare provider on a regular basis to have your health checked and have your diet adjusted as necessary. If you already have any health issues, this is really crucial.

11. Educate Yourself: - Continue to learn about health and nutrition. Ongoing education gives you the ability to make wise decisions and modify your way of life as necessary.

12. Set Achievable and reasonable objectives: - Make reasonable and attainable objectives for your weight loss and general well-being. Acknowledge that improvement is gradual and rejoice in little accomplishments.

13. Innovation in Cooking: - In the kitchen, use your imagination to create tasty and engaging meals. Within the confines of the Atkins diet, try out different dishes and tastes.

14. Create a Support Network: - Create a network of people who are sticking to the same diet, whether it be friends, family, or a community. Support may serve as a source of inspiration and drive.

Preserving Your Success Over Time

Sustaining your progress over time with the Atkins method requires an ongoing dedication to a healthy and balanced way of living. These are some essential tactics to help you maintain your achievements:

1. Regularity in Eating Patterns: - Keep adhering to the Atkins diet guidelines that have helped you succeed. Maintaining a balanced intake of macronutrients and practicing portion control when eating is essential.

2. Consistently Tracking Your Carbohydrate Intake: Remain aware of how much carbohydrates you consume. Keep a close eye on the kinds and quantities of carbs you eat to make sure they support your maintenance objectives.

3. Modify Carbohydrate Levels as Necessary: - Over time, your tolerance for carbohydrates may vary. Be

willing to change your carbohydrate intake in accordance with your unique needs and objectives.

4. Portion Control and Mindful Eating: - Make mindful eating and portion control a habit. To prevent overindulging and preserve a positive connection with food, pay attention to signs of hunger and fullness.

5. Engaging in Regular Exercise: - Include frequent physical exercise in your daily routine. Maintaining a healthy weight, general well-being, and metabolic health are all enhanced by exercise.

6. Hydration and Healthful Behaviors: - Keep giving proper hydration and other healthful behaviors a top priority. Maintaining your accomplishments depends on drinking enough of water, getting enough sleep, and learning how to handle stress.

7. Diversify Your Diet: - Make sure that your diet is rich in nutrients and varied. Include a range of entire meals to guarantee you get a wide range of vital nutrients.

8. Frequent Health Check-Ups: Arrange for routine check-ups to keep an eye on your general health and take care of any new issues that may arise. Making educated judgments about your nutrition and lifestyle might be aided by regular evaluations.

9. Honor Non-Scale Achievements: Celebrate and acknowledge non-scale accomplishments like more energy, a happier mood, or better fitness. These beneficial adjustments support long-term well-being.

10. Evaluate Objectives Reevaluate your weight loss and health objectives on a regular basis. Modify them in

accordance with your lifestyle, present priorities, and general well-being.

11. Create or Maintain a Support Network: - Connect with people who understand and support your health objectives by sharing your experience. Long-term success may greatly benefit from community support.

12. Lifelong Learning and Adaptation: - Remain receptive to further education on wellbeing, health, and nutrition. As your lifestyle, tastes, and health change, adjust your strategy accordingly.

13. Mindful pleasures: - Permit moderation when it comes to mindful pleasures. A sustainable and balanced approach to eating is facilitated by indulging in sweets sometimes and doing so with awareness.

14. Positive Mentality: - Have a positive outlook on your path to better health. Consider the strides you've already achieved and tackle obstacles with resiliency and hope.

Chapter 8
110 Delicious Atkins Recipes

Breakfasts

Egg and Avocado Breakfast Bowl

Prep Time: 10 minutes
Cook Time: 5 minutes
Total Time: 15 minutes
Servings: 2

Ingredients:

- 2 large eggs
- 1 ripe avocado, sliced
- 1 cup cherry tomatoes, halved
- 1/4 cup red onion, finely diced
- 2 tablespoons fresh cilantro, chopped
- 1 tablespoon lime juice
- Salt and pepper to taste
- Optional: hot sauce for added kick

Instructions:

1. Prepare the Eggs:
   - In a medium-sized skillet, heat a bit of cooking spray or olive oil over medium heat.
   - Crack the eggs into the skillet, ensuring the yolks remain intact. Season with salt and pepper.

- Cook the eggs to your preference (fried, poached, or scrambled).

2. Assemble the Bowl:
   - Divide the sliced avocado between two bowls.
   - Place the cooked eggs on top of the avocado.

3. Add Fresh Ingredients:
   - Sprinkle the halved cherry tomatoes and finely diced red onion over the eggs.

4. Enhance with Flavor:
   - Drizzle lime juice over the entire bowl to add a burst of freshness.
   - Sprinkle fresh cilantro on top for added flavor.

5. Optional: Spice it Up:
   - If you enjoy some heat, add a few dashes of your favorite hot sauce.

6. Serve and Enjoy:
   - Serve the Egg and Avocado Breakfast Bowl immediately while the eggs are warm.

Nutritional Information (per serving):

- Calories: 280 kcal
- Protein: 12g
- Fat: 22g
- Carbohydrates: 12g
- Fiber: 7g

Note: Nutritional information is approximate and may vary based on specific ingredients used.

Bacon and Spinach Omelette

Prep Time: 10 minutes
Cook Time: 5 minutes
Total Time: 15 minutes
Servings: 1

Ingredients:

- 2 large eggs
- 2 slices of bacon, cooked and crumbled
- 1 cup fresh spinach leaves, chopped
- 1/4 cup shredded cheddar cheese
- 1/4 cup onion, finely chopped
- 1 tablespoon butter
- Salt and pepper to taste
- Fresh chives for garnish (optional)

Instructions:

1. Cook Bacon:
   - In a skillet over medium heat, cook the bacon until crispy. Remove from the skillet, let it cool, and crumble it.

2. Prepare Spinach:
   - In the same skillet, add chopped spinach and sauté until wilted. Set aside.

3. Whisk Eggs:
   - Crack the eggs into a bowl, add a pinch of salt and pepper, and whisk until well combined.

4. Sauté Onions:
   - In the skillet, sauté chopped onions in butter until they are translucent and fragrant.

5. Cook the Omelette:
   - Pour the whisked eggs over the sautéed onions. Swirl the pan to spread the eggs evenly.
   - As the edges start to set, lift them slightly to allow the uncooked eggs to flow underneath.

6. Add Fillings:
   - Sprinkle crumbled bacon, sautéed spinach, and shredded cheddar cheese on one side of the omelette.

7. Fold and Serve:
   - Once the eggs are fully set but still moist, fold the omelette in half using a spatula.
   - Slide the omelette onto a plate and garnish with fresh chives if desired.

Nutritional Information:
   - Calories: 450 kcal
   - Protein: 26g
   - Fat: 36g
   - Carbohydrates: 5g
   - Fiber: 2g

Note: Nutritional information is approximate and may vary based on specific ingredients used.

Chia Seed Pudding with Berries

Prep Time: 5 minutes (plus overnight chilling)
Total Time: 5 minutes (plus overnight chilling)
Servings: 2

Ingredients:

- 1/4 cup chia seeds
- 1 cup almond milk (or any preferred milk)
- 1 tablespoon maple syrup (adjust to taste)
- 1/2 teaspoon vanilla extract
- A pinch of salt
- 1/2 cup mixed berries (strawberries, blueberries, raspberries)
- 2 tablespoons sliced almonds (optional, for garnish)
- Fresh mint leaves for garnish (optional)

Instructions:

1. Mix Chia Seed Base:
   - In a bowl, combine chia seeds, almond milk, maple syrup, vanilla extract, and a pinch of salt. Stir well to ensure the chia seeds are evenly distributed.

2. Refrigerate Overnight:
   - Cover the bowl and refrigerate the chia seed mixture overnight or for at least 4 hours. This

allows the chia seeds to absorb the liquid and create a pudding-like consistency.

3. Stir Before Serving:
   - Before serving, give the chia seed pudding a good stir to break up any clumps and ensure a smooth texture.

4. Assemble the Pudding Cups:
   - Divide the chia seed pudding into two serving cups or bowls.

5. Top with Berries:
   - Wash and prepare the mixed berries. Spoon them over the chia seed pudding.

6. Garnish:
   - If desired, garnish with sliced almonds for crunch and fresh mint leaves for a burst of freshness.

Nutritional Information (per serving):

   - Calories: 180 kcal
   - Protein: 4g
   - Fat: 8g
   - Carbohydrates: 22g
   - Fiber: 10g

Note: Nutritional information is approximate and may vary based on specific ingredients used.

Sausage and Cheese Breakfast Casserole

Prep Time: 15 minutes
Cook Time: 35 minutes
Total Time: 50 minutes
Servings: 8

Ingredients:

- 1 pound breakfast sausage, cooked and crumbled
- 6 large eggs
- 2 cups milk
- 1 teaspoon Dijon mustard
- 1/2 teaspoon salt
- 1/4 teaspoon black pepper
- 6 cups bread cubes (day-old bread works well)
- 2 cups shredded cheddar cheese
- 1/2 cup diced green bell pepper
- 1/2 cup diced red bell pepper
- 1/4 cup diced onion
- Cooking spray for greasing

Instructions:

1. Preheat Oven:
   - Preheat the oven to 350°F (175°C). Grease a 9x13-inch baking dish with cooking spray.

2. Cook Sausage:

- In a skillet over medium heat, cook the breakfast sausage until browned and crumbled. Drain excess grease and set aside.

3. Prepare Bread Cubes:
    - Cut the bread into cubes, and spread them evenly in the prepared baking dish.

4. Layer Sausage and Vegetables:
    - Sprinkle the cooked sausage over the bread cubes.
    - In a bowl, mix the diced green and red bell peppers, and onion. Spread the vegetable mixture over the sausage.

5. Add Cheese:
    - Sprinkle shredded cheddar cheese evenly over the vegetables and sausage.

6. Prepare Egg Mixture:
    - In a separate bowl, whisk together eggs, milk, Dijon mustard, salt, and black pepper until well combined.

7. Pour Egg Mixture:
    - Pour the egg mixture over the layered ingredients in the baking dish, ensuring even coverage.

8. Bake:
    - Bake in the preheated oven for 35-40 minutes or until the eggs are set and the top is golden brown.

9. Cool and Serve:
   - Allow the casserole to cool for a few minutes before slicing.
   - Serve warm, and enjoy a hearty Sausage and Cheese Breakfast Casserole!

Nutritional Information (per serving):

- Calories: 380 kcal
- Protein: 20g
- Fat: 24g
- Carbohydrates: 22g
- Fiber: 2g

Note: Nutritional information is approximate and may vary based on specific ingredients used.

Smoked Salmon and Cream Cheese Wrap

Prep Time: 10 minutes
Total Time: 10 minutes
Servings: 2

Ingredients:

- 4 ounces smoked salmon
- 4 tablespoons cream cheese, softened
- 2 whole wheat or spinach tortillas (10-inch diameter)
- 1/4 red onion, thinly sliced
- 1/2 cucumber, julienned
- 2 tablespoons capers
- Fresh dill for garnish
- Lemon wedges for serving

Instructions:

1. Prepare Ingredients:
   - Ensure the cream cheese is softened and ready for spreading.
   - Thinly slice the red onion, julienne the cucumber, and gather the capers.

2. Assemble the Wraps:
   - Lay out the tortillas on a clean surface.
   - Spread 2 tablespoons of softened cream cheese onto each tortilla, covering the surface evenly.

3. Layer with Smoked Salmon:
   - Place 2 ounces of smoked salmon on each tortilla, covering the cream cheese.

4. Add Fresh Ingredients:
   - Sprinkle the thinly sliced red onion and julienned cucumber evenly over the smoked salmon.

5. Garnish with Capers and Dill:
   - Sprinkle capers over the wraps for a burst of briny flavor.
   - Garnish with fresh dill for added herbaceousness.

6. Roll the Wraps:
   - Carefully roll up each tortilla into a tight wrap, ensuring the ingredients are well-contained.

7. Slice and Serve:
   - Slice each wrap in half diagonally for easy serving.
   - Serve the Smoked Salmon and Cream Cheese Wraps with lemon wedges on the side.

Nutritional Information (per serving):

- Calories: 320 kcal
- Protein: 18g
- Fat: 18g
- Carbohydrates: 20g
- Fiber: 3g

Note: Nutritional information is approximate and may vary based on specific ingredients used.

Mushroom and Feta Frittata

Prep Time: 15 minutes
Cook Time: 20 minutes
Total Time: 35 minutes
Servings: 4

Ingredients:

- 8 large eggs
- 1 cup mushrooms, sliced
- 1/2 cup crumbled feta cheese
- 1/2 cup cherry tomatoes, halved
- 1/4 cup red onion, finely chopped
- 2 cloves garlic, minced
- 2 tablespoons fresh parsley, chopped
- 1 tablespoon olive oil
- Salt and pepper to taste

Instructions:

1. Preheat Oven:
   - Preheat the oven to 350°F (175°C).

2. Saute Mushrooms:
   - In an oven-safe skillet, heat olive oil over medium heat. Add sliced mushrooms and sauté until they release their moisture and become golden brown. Add minced garlic during the last minute of cooking.

3. Prepare Filling:

- In a bowl, whisk together eggs, salt, and pepper. Stir in crumbled feta, chopped parsley, and finely chopped red onion.

4. Combine Ingredients:
   - Pour the egg mixture over the sautéed mushrooms in the skillet. Gently stir to distribute the ingredients evenly.

5. Add Cherry Tomatoes:
   - Place halved cherry tomatoes on top of the egg mixture.

6. Cook on Stovetop:
   - Cook on the stovetop over medium heat for 3-5 minutes, allowing the edges to set.

7. Transfer to Oven:
   - Transfer the skillet to the preheated oven and bake for 15-18 minutes or until the frittata is set in the center.

8. Serve Warm:
   - Once cooked, remove from the oven and let it cool for a few minutes.
   - Slice the Mushroom and Feta Frittata into wedges and serve warm.

Nutritional Information (per serving):

- Calories: 240 kcal
- Protein: 18g

- Fat: 16g
- Carbohydrates: 6g
- Fiber: 2g

Note: Nutritional information is approximate and may vary based on specific ingredients used.

Low-Carb Yogurt Parfait

Prep Time: 10 minutes
Total Time: 10 minutes
Servings: 2

Ingredients:

- 1 cup Greek yogurt (unsweetened)
- 1/2 cup fresh strawberries, sliced
- 1/4 cup blueberries
- 2 tablespoons almond slices
- 2 tablespoons chia seeds
- 1 teaspoon vanilla extract
- 1 tablespoon sugar-free sweetener (optional)
- Fresh mint leaves for garnish (optional)

Instructions:

1. Prepare Yogurt Base:
   - In a bowl, combine Greek yogurt, vanilla extract, and sugar-free sweetener if desired. Mix well until smooth.

2. Layer Yogurt:
   - Spoon a layer of the yogurt mixture into the bottom of serving glasses or bowls.

3. Add Strawberries:
   - Place a layer of sliced strawberries on top of the yogurt.

4. Sprinkle with Almonds and Chia Seeds:
   - Sprinkle almond slices and chia seeds over the strawberries.

5. Repeat Layers:
   - Repeat the layering process by adding another layer of yogurt, followed by blueberries.

6. Top with Fresh Mint (Optional):
   - Garnish the top with fresh mint leaves for a burst of freshness.

7. Serve Immediately:
   - Serve the Low-Carb Yogurt Parfait immediately, or refrigerate for a chilled treat.

 Nutritional Information (per serving):

- Calories: 200 kcal
- Protein: 15g
- Fat: 10g
- Carbohydrates: 15g
- Fiber: 6g

Note: Nutritional information is approximate and may vary based on specific ingredients used.

Keto Pancakes with Sugar-Free Syrup

Prep Time: 10 minutes
Cook Time: 10 minutes
Total Time: 20 minutes
Servings: 2 (4-5 pancakes each)

Pancake Ingredients:

- 1 cup almond flour
- 2 tablespoons coconut flour
- 2 teaspoons baking powder
- 3 large eggs
- 1/2 cup unsweetened almond milk
- 2 tablespoons melted butter or coconut oil
- 1 teaspoon vanilla extract
- 1-2 tablespoons sugar-free sweetener (to taste)
- Pinch of salt

Sugar-Free Syrup Ingredients:

- 1/2 cup water
- 1/2 cup sugar-free sweetener
- 1 teaspoon vanilla extract
- 1/2 teaspoon xanthan gum (optional, for thickness)

Instructions:

Keto Pancakes:

1. Prepare Dry Ingredients:

- In a mixing bowl, whisk together almond flour, coconut flour, baking powder, sugar-free sweetener, and a pinch of salt.

2. Combine Wet Ingredients:
   - In a separate bowl, beat the eggs. Add almond milk, melted butter or coconut oil, and vanilla extract. Mix well.

3. Combine Wet and Dry Ingredients:
   - Pour the wet ingredients into the dry ingredients and stir until just combined. Let the batter rest for a few minutes to allow the coconut flour to absorb the liquids.

4. Cook Pancakes:
   - Heat a griddle or non-stick skillet over medium heat. Grease with butter or oil.
   - Spoon the batter onto the hot griddle to form pancakes. Cook until bubbles form on the surface, then flip and cook the other side until golden brown.

5. Serve Warm:
   - Stack the keto pancakes and keep them warm until ready to serve.

 Sugar-Free Syrup:

1. Combine Ingredients:
   - In a small saucepan, combine water, sugar-free sweetener, and vanilla extract. Bring to a simmer over medium heat.

2. Optional Thickening:
   - If desired, sprinkle xanthan gum over the simmering syrup and whisk continuously to avoid lumps. Continue to simmer until the syrup thickens to your liking.

3. Cool and Serve:
   - Remove the syrup from heat and let it cool slightly before serving.

 Nutritional Information (per serving - 2 pancakes with syrup):

- Calories: 400 kcal
- Protein: 15g
- Fat: 32g
- Carbohydrates: 12g
- Fiber: 6g

Note: Nutritional information is approximate and may vary based on specific ingredients used.

Vegetable and Ham Egg Muffins

Prep Time: 15 minutes
Cook Time: 20 minutes
Total Time: 35 minutes
Servings: 6

Ingredients:

- 8 large eggs
- 1/2 cup diced ham
- 1/2 cup bell peppers, finely diced (mix of colors)
- 1/2 cup cherry tomatoes, diced
- 1/4 cup red onion, finely chopped
- 1/4 cup spinach, chopped
- 1/4 cup shredded cheddar cheese
- 2 tablespoons milk or unsweetened almond milk
- 1 tablespoon olive oil
- 1 teaspoon dried oregano
- Salt and pepper to taste

Instructions:

1. Preheat Oven:
   - Preheat the oven to 350°F (175°C). Grease a muffin tin with cooking spray or use silicone muffin cups.

2. Prepare Vegetables:
   - In a skillet, heat olive oil over medium heat. Add diced ham, bell peppers, cherry tomatoes, red

onion, and spinach. Sauté for 3-4 minutes until the vegetables are slightly softened. Set aside to cool.

3. Whisk Eggs:
    - In a bowl, whisk together eggs, milk, dried oregano, salt, and pepper until well combined.

4. Combine Ingredients:
    - Add the sautéed vegetables and shredded cheddar cheese to the egg mixture. Mix well.

5. Fill Muffin Cups:
    - Pour the egg and vegetable mixture evenly into the muffin cups, filling each cup about three-quarters full.

6. Bake:
    - Bake in the preheated oven for 18-20 minutes or until the tops are set and slightly golden.

7. Cool and Serve:
    - Allow the Vegetable and Ham Egg Muffins to cool in the muffin tin for a few minutes before transferring them to a wire rack.

Nutritional Information (per serving - 2 muffins):

- Calories: 220 kcal
- Protein: 18g
- Fat: 14g
- Carbohydrates: 5g
- Fiber: 1g

Note: Nutritional information is approximate and may vary based on specific ingredients used.

Avocado and Bacon Breakfast Wrap

Prep Time: 15 minutes
Cook Time: 10 minutes
Total Time: 25 minutes
Servings: 2

Ingredients:

- 4 slices of bacon
- 2 large eggs
- 1 ripe avocado, sliced
- 1 medium tomato, sliced
- 2 whole wheat or low-carb tortillas
- 1/4 cup shredded cheddar cheese
- Salt and pepper to taste
- Fresh cilantro for garnish (optional)
- Hot sauce for drizzling (optional)

Instructions:

1. Cook Bacon:
   - In a skillet over medium heat, cook the bacon until crispy. Remove and drain on paper towels.

2. Scramble Eggs:
   - In the same skillet, pour out excess bacon grease, leaving about a teaspoon in the pan. Crack the eggs into the skillet, scramble, and cook until just set. Season with salt and pepper.

3. Warm Tortillas:

- Heat the tortillas in the skillet or microwave according to package instructions.

4. Assemble Wraps:
   - Lay out the warm tortillas on a clean surface.
   - Divide the scrambled eggs between the tortillas, placing them in the center.

5. Layer with Ingredients:
   - Add sliced avocado, tomato slices, and crispy bacon on top of the eggs.

6. Sprinkle with Cheese:
   - Sprinkle shredded cheddar cheese over the ingredients on each tortilla.

7. Fold and Serve:
   - Carefully fold the sides of the tortillas and roll them into wraps.

8. Garnish and Drizzle (Optional):
   - Garnish with fresh cilantro and drizzle with hot sauce if desired.

9. Serve Immediately:
   - Serve the Avocado and Bacon Breakfast Wraps immediately while warm.

Nutritional Information (per serving):

- Calories: 450 kcal
- Protein: 20g
- Fat: 32g

- Carbohydrates: 24g
- Fiber: 8g

Note: Nutritional information is approximate and may vary based on specific ingredients used.

Coconut Flour Porridge with Almonds

Prep Time: 5 minutes
Cook Time: 10 minutes
Total Time: 15 minutes
Servings: 2

Ingredients:

- 1/2 cup coconut flour
- 2 cups unsweetened almond milk
- 2 tablespoons coconut oil
- 2 tablespoons shredded coconut (unsweetened)
- 2 tablespoons almond butter
- 1/4 cup sliced almonds
- 1 teaspoon vanilla extract
- 1-2 tablespoons sugar-free sweetener (to taste)
- Pinch of salt
- Fresh berries for topping (optional)

Instructions:

1. Mix Dry Ingredients:
   - In a bowl, combine coconut flour, shredded coconut, sliced almonds, and a pinch of salt.

2. Heat Almond Milk:
   - In a saucepan, heat almond milk over medium heat until it starts to simmer.

3. Combine Wet Ingredients:

- In a separate bowl, mix together coconut oil, almond butter, and vanilla extract.

4. Create Porridge Base:
   - Add the dry ingredients to the simmering almond milk, stirring continuously to avoid lumps.

5. Add Wet Ingredients:
   - Pour in the coconut oil, almond butter, and vanilla extract mixture. Continue stirring until the porridge thickens.

6. Sweeten to Taste:
   - Add sugar-free sweetener to taste. Stir well to incorporate.

7. Serve Warm:
   - Once the porridge reaches your desired consistency, remove from heat.

8. Top with Almonds and Berries:
   - Divide the porridge into bowls. Top with sliced almonds and fresh berries if desired.

9. Serve Immediately:
   - Serve the Coconut Flour Porridge with Almonds warm.

Nutritional Information (per serving):

- Calories: 380 kcal
- Protein: 10g
- Fat: 30g

- Carbohydrates: 18g
- Fiber: 12g

Note: Nutritional information is approximate and may vary based on specific ingredients used.

Turkey and Cheese Roll-Ups

Prep Time: 10 minutes
Total Time: 10 minutes
Servings: 2

Ingredients:

- 8 slices of roasted turkey breast (thinly sliced)
- 4 slices of your favorite cheese (cheddar, Swiss, or pepper jack work well)
- 1/2 cup baby spinach leaves
- 1/4 cup mayonnaise
- 1 tablespoon Dijon mustard
- Salt and pepper to taste
- Toothpicks for securing

Instructions:

1. Prepare **Ingredients:**
   - Lay out the turkey slices on a clean surface.
   - In a small bowl, mix mayonnaise and Dijon mustard.

2. Spread Sauce:
   - Spread a thin layer of the mayonnaise and Dijon mixture over each turkey slice.

3. Layer with Cheese and Spinach:
   - Place a slice of cheese on top of the sauce-covered turkey.

- Add a handful of baby spinach leaves on top of the cheese.

4. Roll Up:
 - Starting from one end, tightly roll up each turkey slice with the cheese and spinach inside.

5. Secure with Toothpicks:
 - Use toothpicks to secure the ends of the turkey roll-ups, ensuring they hold their shape.

6. Slice and Serve:
 - With a sharp knife, slice each roll-up into bite-sized pieces.

7. Serve Cold:
 - Serve the Turkey and Cheese Roll-Ups cold as a quick and satisfying snack or appetizer.

 Nutritional Information (per serving):

- Calories: 320 kcal
- Protein: 25g
- Fat: 22g
- Carbohydrates: 2g
- Fiber: 1g

Note: Nutritional information is approximate and may vary based on specific ingredients used.

Low-Carb Breakfast Burrito

Prep Time: 15 minutes
Cook Time: 10 minutes
Total Time: 25 minutes
Servings: 2

Ingredients:

- 4 large eggs
- 1 tablespoon olive oil
- 1/2 bell pepper, diced
- 1/2 small onion, finely chopped
- 2 cloves garlic, minced
- 4 slices turkey or chicken bacon
- 4 low-carb tortillas (8-inch diameter)
- 1/2 cup shredded cheddar cheese
- 1 medium avocado, sliced
- Salt and pepper to taste
- Hot sauce or salsa for serving (optional)
- Fresh cilantro for garnish (optional)

Instructions:

1. Cook Bacon:
   - In a skillet over medium heat, cook the turkey or chicken bacon until crispy. Remove and drain on paper towels. Chop into small pieces.

2. Saute Vegetables:

- In the same skillet, add olive oil and sauté diced bell pepper, chopped onion, and minced garlic until softened.

3. Scramble Eggs:
   - Push the sautéed vegetables to one side of the skillet. Crack the eggs into the empty side, season with salt and pepper, and scramble until just set.

4. Combine Ingredients:
   - Mix the scrambled eggs with the sautéed vegetables and add the chopped bacon. Stir until well combined.

5. Warm Tortillas:
   - Heat the low-carb tortillas in the skillet or microwave according to package instructions.

6. Assemble Burritos:
   - Divide the egg and vegetable mixture evenly among the tortillas.
   - Top each with shredded cheddar cheese and slices of avocado.

7. Fold and Serve:
   - Fold the sides of each tortilla and roll them into burritos.

8. Serve Warm:
   - Serve the Low-Carb Breakfast Burritos immediately while warm.

Nutritional Information (per serving):

- Calories: 480 kcal
- Protein: 24g
- Fat: 36g
- Carbohydrates: 18g
- Fiber: 10g

Note: Nutritional information is approximate and may vary based on specific ingredients used.

Cauliflower Hash Browns

Prep Time: 15 minutes
Cook Time: 20 minutes
Total Time: 35 minutes
Servings: 4

Ingredients:

- 1 medium cauliflower head, grated or riced
- 2 large eggs
- 1/4 cup almond flour
- 1/4 cup grated Parmesan cheese
- 1/2 teaspoon garlic powder
- 1/2 teaspoon onion powder
- 1/2 teaspoon paprika
- Salt and pepper to taste
- Cooking spray or olive oil for frying

Instructions:

1. Prepare Cauliflower:
   - Grate the cauliflower using a box grater or pulse it in a food processor until it resembles rice.

2. Drain Excess Moisture:
   - Place the grated cauliflower in a clean kitchen towel or cheesecloth and squeeze out any excess moisture.

3. Combine Ingredients:

- In a large bowl, combine the grated cauliflower, eggs, almond flour, Parmesan cheese, garlic powder, onion powder, paprika, salt, and pepper. Mix well until all ingredients are evenly combined.

4. Form Hash Browns:
   - Divide the mixture into equal portions and shape them into round patties, similar to traditional hash browns.

5. Cook on Skillet:
   - Heat a skillet over medium heat and coat it with cooking spray or olive oil.
   - Cook the cauliflower hash browns for 3-4 minutes on each side or until they are golden brown and cooked through.

6. Serve Warm:
   - Remove from the skillet and place on a plate lined with a paper towel to absorb any excess oil.
   - Serve the Cauliflower Hash Browns warm.

Nutritional Information (per serving - 2 hash browns):

- Calories: 120 kcal
- Protein: 8g
- Fat: 7g
- Carbohydrates: 9g
- Fiber: 3g

Note: Nutritional information is approximate and may vary based on specific ingredients used.

Spinach and Feta Breakfast Muffins

Prep Time: 15 minutes
Cook Time: 20 minutes
Total Time: 35 minutes
Servings: 12 muffins

Ingredients:

- 2 cups fresh spinach, chopped
- 1/2 cup red bell pepper, diced
- 1/4 cup red onion, finely chopped
- 1 cup feta cheese, crumbled
- 8 large eggs
- 1/2 cup milk (dairy or plant-based)
- 1 teaspoon olive oil
- 1 teaspoon dried oregano
- Salt and pepper to taste
- Cooking spray for muffin tin

Instructions:

1. Preheat Oven:
   - Preheat the oven to 375°F (190°C). Grease a muffin tin with cooking spray.

2. Saute Vegetables:
   - In a skillet over medium heat, sauté chopped spinach, diced red bell pepper, and finely chopped red onion in olive oil until the vegetables are softened. Allow them to cool.

3. Prepare Egg Mixture:
   - In a large bowl, whisk together eggs and milk. Add crumbled feta, dried oregano, salt, and pepper. Mix well.

4. Add Sauteed Vegetables:
   - Fold the sautéed spinach, red bell pepper, and red onion into the egg mixture.

5. Fill Muffin Tin:
   - Pour the mixture evenly into the greased muffin tin.

6. Bake:
   - Bake in the preheated oven for 20-25 minutes or until the muffins are set and the tops are golden brown.

7. Cool and Serve:
   - Allow the Spinach and Feta Breakfast Muffins to cool for a few minutes in the tin before transferring them to a wire rack to cool completely.

8. Serve Warm or Cold:
   - Serve the muffins warm or cold. They can be stored in an airtight container in the refrigerator for up to a week.

Nutritional Information (per muffin):

- Calories: 120 kcal

- Protein: 8g
- Fat: 8g
- Carbohydrates: 3g
- Fiber: 1g

Note: Nutritional information is approximate and may vary based on specific ingredients used.

Keto Avocado Smoothie

Prep Time: 5 minutes
Total Time: 5 minutes
Servings: 2

Ingredients:

- 1 ripe avocado, peeled and pitted
- 1 cup unsweetened almond milk
- 1/2 cup full-fat Greek yogurt
- 2 tablespoons chia seeds
- 1 tablespoon almond butter
- 1-2 tablespoons sugar-free sweetener (to taste)
- 1 teaspoon vanilla extract
- Ice cubes (optional)
- Fresh mint leaves for garnish (optional)

Instructions:

1. Prepare Avocado:
   - Cut the ripe avocado in half, remove the pit, and scoop out the flesh.

2. Combine Ingredients:
   - In a blender, combine the avocado, almond milk, Greek yogurt, chia seeds, almond butter, sugar-free sweetener, and vanilla extract.

3. Blend Until Smooth:

- Blend the ingredients until the mixture is smooth and creamy. Add ice cubes if you prefer a colder smoothie.

4. Taste and Adjust:
   - Taste the smoothie and adjust the sweetness by adding more sugar-free sweetener if needed.

5. Serve:
   - Pour the Keto Avocado Smoothie into glasses.

6. Garnish (Optional):
   - Garnish with fresh mint leaves for a burst of freshness.

7. Serve Immediately:
   - Serve the smoothie immediately for the best texture and flavor.

Nutritional Information (per serving):

- Calories: 220 kcal
- Protein: 8g
- Fat: 18g
- Carbohydrates: 8g
- Fiber: 6g

Note: Nutritional information is approximate and may vary based on specific ingredients used.

Caprese Egg Bake

Prep Time: 15 minutes
Cook Time: 25 minutes
Total Time: 40 minutes
Servings: 4

Ingredients:

- 8 large eggs
- 1 cup cherry tomatoes, halved
- 1 cup fresh mozzarella, diced
- 1/4 cup fresh basil, chopped
- 2 tablespoons balsamic glaze
- 1 tablespoon olive oil
- Salt and pepper to taste
- Cooking spray for baking dish

Instructions:

1. Preheat Oven:
    - Preheat the oven to 375°F (190°C). Grease a baking dish with cooking spray.

2. Prepare Eggs:
    - Crack the eggs into a bowl, season with salt and pepper, and beat them until well combined.

3. Layer Ingredients:
    - Pour the beaten eggs into the greased baking dish.

- Scatter halved cherry tomatoes, diced fresh mozzarella, and chopped fresh basil evenly over the eggs.

4. Drizzle with Balsamic Glaze:
   - Drizzle balsamic glaze and olive oil over the ingredients.

5. Bake:
   - Bake in the preheated oven for 20-25 minutes or until the eggs are set and the top is golden brown.

6. Cool and Slice:
   - Allow the Caprese Egg Bake to cool for a few minutes before slicing it into squares or wedges.

7. Serve Warm:
   - Serve the egg bake warm, garnished with additional fresh basil if desired.

Nutritional Information (per serving):

- Calories: 240 kcal
- Protein: 18g
- Fat: 16g
- Carbohydrates: 6g
- Fiber: 1g

Note: Nutritional information is approximate and may vary based on specific ingredients used.

Almond Flour Waffles

Prep Time: 10 minutes
Cook Time: 10 minutes
Total Time: 20 minutes
Servings: 4 (2 waffles per serving)

Ingredients:

- 2 cups almond flour
- 4 large eggs
- 1/2 cup unsweetened almond milk
- 1/4 cup melted butter or coconut oil
- 2 tablespoons sugar-free sweetener (optional)
- 1 teaspoon baking powder
- 1/2 teaspoon vanilla extract
- Pinch of salt
- Cooking spray for waffle iron

Instructions:

1. Preheat Waffle Iron:
    - Preheat your waffle iron according to the manufacturer's instructions.

2. Mix Dry Ingredients:
    - In a large bowl, whisk together almond flour, baking powder, sugar-free sweetener (if using), and a pinch of salt.

3. Combine Wet Ingredients:

- In a separate bowl, beat the eggs. Add melted butter or coconut oil, unsweetened almond milk, and vanilla extract. Mix well.

4. Create Batter:
   - Pour the wet ingredients into the dry ingredients and stir until a thick batter forms.

5. Grease Waffle Iron:
   - Lightly grease the preheated waffle iron with cooking spray.

6. Cook Waffles:
   - Spoon the batter onto the center of the waffle iron, spreading it slightly. Close the lid and cook until the waffles are golden brown and crisp.

7. Serve Warm:
   - Carefully remove the waffles from the iron and serve them warm.

Nutritional Information (per serving - 2 waffles):

- Calories: 400 kcal
- Protein: 14g
- Fat: 34g
- Carbohydrates: 10g
- Fiber: 4g

Note: Nutritional information is approximate and may vary based on specific ingredients used.

Greek Yogurt Breakfast Bowl

Prep Time: 5 minutes
Total Time: 5 minutes
Servings: 1

Ingredients:

- 1 cup Greek yogurt (unsweetened)
- 1/2 cup mixed berries (blueberries, strawberries, raspberries)
- 1/4 cup granola (sugar-free for a low-carb option)
- 1 tablespoon chia seeds
- 1 tablespoon honey or sugar-free sweetener (optional)
- 1 tablespoon chopped nuts (almonds, walnuts, or pistachios)
- Fresh mint leaves for garnish (optional)

Instructions:

1. Prepare Greek Yogurt Base:
   - Spoon Greek yogurt into a bowl, spreading it evenly.

2. Add Mixed Berries:
   - Scatter mixed berries over the Greek yogurt.

3. Sprinkle Granola:
   - Sprinkle granola over the berries, adding a satisfying crunch.

4. Top with Chia Seeds:
   - Sprinkle chia seeds over the granola for added fiber and texture.

5. Drizzle with Honey (Optional):
   - If desired, drizzle honey or a sugar-free sweetener over the top for added sweetness.

6. Garnish with Nuts:
   - Sprinkle chopped nuts over the bowl for a boost of healthy fats.

7. Garnish with Mint (Optional):
   - Garnish with fresh mint leaves for a burst of freshness.

8. Serve Immediately:
   - Serve the Greek Yogurt Breakfast Bowl immediately and enjoy the nutritious and delicious combination of flavors and textures.

Nutritional Information:

- Calories: 350 kcal
- Protein: 20g
- Fat: 15g
- Carbohydrates: 40g
- Fiber: 8g

Note: Nutritional information is approximate and may vary based on specific ingredients used.

Zucchini and Cheese Fritters

Prep Time: 15 minutes
Cook Time: 15 minutes
Total Time: 30 minutes
Servings: 4

Ingredients:

- 2 medium zucchinis, grated
- 1 cup shredded cheddar cheese
- 1/4 cup grated Parmesan cheese
- 1/4 cup almond flour
- 2 large eggs
- 2 tablespoons chopped fresh parsley
- 1 clove garlic, minced
- 1/2 teaspoon onion powder
- Salt and pepper to taste
- Cooking oil for frying (olive oil or avocado oil)

Instructions:

1. Prepare Zucchinis:
   - Grate the zucchinis using a box grater or a food processor. Place the grated zucchini in a clean kitchen towel and squeeze out excess moisture.

2. Combine Ingredients:
   - In a large bowl, combine the grated zucchini, shredded cheddar cheese, Parmesan cheese, almond flour, eggs, chopped parsley, minced garlic,

onion powder, salt, and pepper. Mix well until all ingredients are evenly incorporated.

3. Form Fritters:
   - Scoop a portion of the mixture and shape it into a small patty, forming fritters with your hands.

4. Heat Cooking Oil:
   - Heat cooking oil in a skillet over medium heat.

5. Fry Fritters:
   - Carefully place the fritters in the hot oil, cooking for 3-4 minutes on each side or until they are golden brown and crispy.

6. Drain Excess Oil:
   - Place the cooked fritters on a plate lined with paper towels to drain any excess oil.

7. Serve Warm:
   - Serve the Zucchini and Cheese Fritters warm, optionally garnished with additional chopped parsley.

Nutritional Information (per serving):

- Calories: 220 kcal
- Protein: 12g
- Fat: 16g
- Carbohydrates: 8g
- Fiber: 3g

Note: Nutritional information is approximate and may vary based on specific ingredients used.

Creamy Mushroom and Spinach Scramble

Prep Time: 10 minutes
Cook Time: 10 minutes
Total Time: 20 minutes
Servings: 2

Ingredients:

- 4 large eggs
- 1 cup mushrooms, sliced
- 2 cups fresh spinach leaves
- 1/2 cup heavy cream
- 1/4 cup grated Parmesan cheese
- 2 tablespoons butter
- 2 cloves garlic, minced
- 1/2 teaspoon dried thyme
- Salt and pepper to taste
- Fresh parsley for garnish (optional)

Instructions:

1. Whisk Eggs:
   - In a bowl, whisk the eggs until well beaten. Add a pinch of salt and pepper to season.

2. Saute Mushrooms:
   - In a skillet, melt 1 tablespoon of butter over medium heat. Add sliced mushrooms and minced garlic. Saute until the mushrooms are golden brown and the garlic is fragrant.

3. Add Spinach:
   - Add fresh spinach to the skillet and cook until wilted.

4. Pour in Cream:
   - Pour in the heavy cream and stir well, allowing it to simmer for a minute.

5. Scramble Eggs:
   - Push the mushroom and spinach mixture to one side of the skillet. Add the remaining tablespoon of butter to the empty side and pour in the beaten eggs. Allow the eggs to set for a moment, then gently scramble them.

6. Combine and Season:
   - Once the eggs are almost fully cooked, mix them with the mushroom and spinach mixture. Add dried thyme, grated Parmesan cheese, and season with salt and pepper to taste.

7. Garnish and Serve:
   - Garnish with fresh parsley if desired. Serve the Creamy Mushroom and Spinach Scramble immediately.

Nutritional Information (per serving):

- Calories: 380 kcal
- Protein: 16g
- Fat: 32g

- Carbohydrates: 6g
- Fiber: 2g

Note: Nutritional information is approximate and may vary based on specific ingredients used.

Creamy Protein-Packed Breakfast Salad

Prep Time: 15 minutes
Cook Time: 10 minutes
Total Time: 25 minutes
Servings: 2

Ingredients:

- 4 large eggs
- 1 cup cherry tomatoes, halved
- 1/2 cucumber, diced
- 1/4 cup red onion, finely chopped
- 1/4 cup feta cheese, crumbled
- 1/4 cup plain Greek yogurt
- 2 tablespoons olive oil
- 1 tablespoon lemon juice
- 1 teaspoon Dijon mustard
- 1 teaspoon honey or sugar-free sweetener
- Salt and pepper to taste
- 2 cups mixed salad greens

Instructions:

1. Boil Eggs:
   - Bring a pot of water to a boil. Carefully add the eggs and boil for 8-10 minutes. Once done, cool the eggs under cold running water, peel, and slice them.

2. Prepare Salad Base:

- In a large bowl, combine the salad greens, halved cherry tomatoes, diced cucumber, finely chopped red onion, and crumbled feta cheese.

3. Make Creamy Dressing:
   - In a small bowl, whisk together Greek yogurt, olive oil, lemon juice, Dijon mustard, honey or sugar-free sweetener, salt, and pepper until well combined.

4. Assemble Salad:
   - Drizzle the creamy dressing over the salad base and toss gently to coat the ingredients evenly.

5. Add Sliced Eggs:
   - Arrange the sliced boiled eggs on top of the salad.

6. Serve:
   - Divide the Creamy Protein-Packed Breakfast Salad into two bowls and serve immediately.

Nutritional Information (per serving):

- Calories: 350 kcal
- Protein: 18g
- Fat: 24g
- Carbohydrates: 15g
- Fiber: 4g

Note: Nutritional information is approximate and may vary based on specific ingredients used.

Baked Avocado Eggs

Prep Time: 10 minutes
Cook Time: 15 minutes
Total Time: 25 minutes
Servings: 2

Ingredients:

- 2 ripe avocados
- 4 large eggs
- Salt and pepper to taste
- 1/4 cup shredded cheddar cheese
- 2 tablespoons chopped fresh chives or parsley (for garnish)
- Hot sauce or salsa (optional, for serving)

Instructions:

1. Preheat Oven:
   - Preheat the oven to 375°F (190°C).

2. Prepare Avocados:
   - Cut the avocados in half, and carefully scoop out a small portion of the flesh to create a well for the eggs.

3. Place Avocados on Baking Sheet:
   - Place the avocado halves on a baking sheet, ensuring they are stable and won't tip over.

4. Crack Eggs into Avocado Wells:

- Crack one egg into each avocado half. Season with salt and pepper to taste.

5. Bake:
  - Bake in the preheated oven for 15-20 minutes or until the egg whites are set but the yolks are still slightly runny.

6. Add Cheese:
  - Sprinkle shredded cheddar cheese over the eggs during the last 5 minutes of baking, allowing it to melt.

7. Garnish and Serve:
    - Remove from the oven and garnish with chopped fresh chives or parsley.

8. Serve Warm:
  - Serve the Baked Avocado Eggs warm, optionally with hot sauce or salsa on the side.

Nutritional Information (per serving - 1 avocado half with 2 eggs):

- Calories: 320 kcal
- Protein: 16g
- Fat: 26g
- Carbohydrates: 12g
- Fiber: 9g

Note: Nutritional information is approximate and may vary based on specific ingredients used.

Keto Blueberry Muffins

Prep Time: 10 minutes
Cook Time: 20 minutes
Total Time: 30 minutes
Servings: 12 muffins

Ingredients:

- 2 cups almond flour
- 1/4 cup coconut flour
- 1/3 cup granulated sugar substitute (e.g., erythritol)
- 1 teaspoon baking powder
- 1/2 teaspoon baking soda
- 1/4 teaspoon salt
- 1/2 cup unsalted butter, melted
- 3 large eggs
- 1/2 cup unsweetened almond milk
- 1 teaspoon vanilla extract
- 1 cup fresh or frozen blueberries

Instructions:

1. Preheat Oven:
   - Preheat the oven to 350°F (175°C). Line a muffin tin with paper liners.

2. Mix Dry Ingredients:
   - In a large bowl, whisk together almond flour, coconut flour, sugar substitute, baking powder, baking soda, and salt.

3. Combine Wet Ingredients:
  - In a separate bowl, whisk together melted butter, eggs, almond milk, and vanilla extract.

4. Combine Wet and Dry Ingredients:
  - Pour the wet ingredients into the dry ingredients and stir until well combined.

5. Fold in Blueberries:
  - Gently fold in the blueberries, being careful not to overmix.

6. Fill Muffin Cups:
  - Spoon the batter into the muffin cups, filling each about two-thirds full.

7. Bake:
  - Bake in the preheated oven for 18-20 minutes or until a toothpick inserted into the center comes out clean.

8. Cool and Serve:
  - Allow the Keto Blueberry Muffins to cool in the tin for a few minutes before transferring them to a wire rack to cool completely.

Nutritional Information (per muffin):

- Calories: 180 kcal
- Protein: 5g
- Fat: 15g

- Carbohydrates: 6g
- Fiber: 3g
- Net Carbs: 3g

Note: Nutritional information is approximate and may vary based on specific ingredients used.

Cottage Cheese and Berry Bowl

Prep Time: 5 minutes
Total Time: 5 minutes
Servings: 2

Ingredients:

- 1 cup low-fat cottage cheese
- 1 cup mixed berries (strawberries, blueberries, raspberries)
- 2 tablespoons chopped nuts (almonds, walnuts, or pistachios)
- 1 tablespoon chia seeds
- 1 tablespoon honey or sugar-free sweetener (optional)
- Fresh mint leaves for garnish (optional)

Instructions:

1. Prepare Cottage Cheese Base:
   - Spoon low-fat cottage cheese into serving bowls.

2. Add Mixed Berries:
   - Scatter mixed berries over the cottage cheese.

3. Sprinkle Nuts:
   - Sprinkle chopped nuts over the berries for added crunch and texture.

4. Top with Chia Seeds:

- Sprinkle chia seeds over the bowl for additional fiber and nutrition.

5. Drizzle with Honey (Optional):
   - If desired, drizzle honey or a sugar-free sweetener over the top for added sweetness.

6. Garnish with Mint (Optional):
   - Garnish the Cottage Cheese and Berry Bowl with fresh mint leaves for a burst of freshness.

7. Serve Immediately:
   - Serve the Cottage Cheese and Berry Bowl immediately, enjoying the delightful combination of creamy cottage cheese and vibrant berries.

Nutritional Information (per serving):

- Calories: 220 kcal
- Protein: 18g
- Fat: 8g
- Carbohydrates: 20g
- Fiber: 5g

Note: Nutritional information is approximate and may vary based on specific ingredients used.

Lunch

Grilled Chicken Caesar Salad

Prep Time: 15 minutes
Cook Time: 15 minutes
Total Time: 30 minutes
Servings: 2

Ingredients:

For Grilled Chicken:

- 2 boneless, skinless chicken breasts
- 2 tablespoons olive oil
- 1 teaspoon garlic powder
- 1 teaspoon dried oregano
- Salt and pepper to taste

For Caesar Salad:

- 1 large head of romaine lettuce, washed and chopped
- 1/2 cup cherry tomatoes, halved
- 1/4 cup grated Parmesan cheese
- 1/4 cup Caesar dressing (store-bought or homemade)
- 1/4 cup croutons (optional)
- Lemon wedges for garnish (optional)

Instructions:

Grilled Chicken:

1. Preheat Grill:
   - Preheat the grill to medium-high heat.

2. Season Chicken:
   - In a bowl, mix olive oil, garlic powder, dried oregano, salt, and pepper. Coat the chicken breasts with this mixture.

3. Grill Chicken:
   - Grill the chicken breasts for 6-8 minutes per side or until the internal temperature reaches 165°F (74°C). Allow the chicken to rest for a few minutes before slicing.

Caesar Salad:

1. Prepare Salad Base:
   - In a large salad bowl, combine chopped romaine lettuce, cherry tomatoes, and grated Parmesan cheese.

2. Add Grilled Chicken:
   - Slice the grilled chicken and add it to the salad.

3. Dress the Salad:
   - Drizzle Caesar dressing over the salad and toss to coat evenly.

4. Optional Croutons:

- If desired, add croutons for added crunch.

5. Garnish and Serve:
    - Garnish with lemon wedges and serve the Grilled Chicken Caesar Salad immediately.

 Nutritional Information (per serving):

- Calories: 450 kcal
- Protein: 35g
- Fat: 28g
- Carbohydrates: 15g
- Fiber: 5g

Note: Nutritional information is approximate and may vary based on specific ingredients used.

Salmon and Avocado Lettuce Wraps

Prep Time: 15 minutes
Cook Time: 10 minutes
Total Time: 25 minutes
Servings: 2

Ingredients:

For Salmon:

- 2 salmon fillets
- 1 tablespoon olive oil
- 1 teaspoon lemon juice
- 1 teaspoon dried dill
- Salt and pepper to taste

For Lettuce Wraps:

- 1 large head of iceberg or butter lettuce, leaves separated
- 1 avocado, sliced
- 1/2 cucumber, julienned
- 1/4 cup red onion, thinly sliced
- 2 tablespoons plain Greek yogurt
- Fresh dill for garnish (optional)

Instructions:

Salmon:

1. Preheat Oven:

  - Preheat the oven to 400°F (200°C).

2. Season Salmon:
   - In a bowl, mix olive oil, lemon juice, dried dill, salt, and pepper. Coat the salmon fillets with this mixture.

3. Bake Salmon:
   - Place the salmon fillets on a baking sheet and bake for 10 minutes or until the salmon flakes easily with a fork.

4. Flake Salmon:
   - Once cooked, flake the salmon into bite-sized pieces.

Lettuce Wraps:

1. Prepare Lettuce Leaves:
   - Wash and separate the leaves of iceberg or butter lettuce.

2. Assemble Wraps:
   - On each lettuce leaf, layer slices of avocado, julienned cucumber, and red onion.

3. Add Salmon:
   - Top the vegetable layers with flaked salmon.

4. Drizzle with Yogurt:
   - Drizzle each wrap with a tablespoon of plain Greek yogurt.

5. Garnish and Serve:
   - Garnish with fresh dill if desired. Serve the Salmon and Avocado Lettuce Wraps immediately.

Nutritional Information (per serving):

- Calories: 350 kcal
- Protein: 25g
- Fat: 20g
- Carbohydrates: 15g
- Fiber: 7g

Note: Nutritional information is approximate and may vary based on specific ingredients used.

Turkey and Bacon Lettuce Cups

Prep Time: 15 minutes
Cook Time: 10 minutes
Total Time: 25 minutes
Servings: 4

Ingredients:

- 1lb ground turkey
- 8 slices bacon, cooked and crumbled
- 1 teaspoon olive oil
- 1 small onion, finely chopped
- 2 cloves garlic, minced
- 1 teaspoon ground cumin
- 1 teaspoon chili powder
- Salt and pepper to taste
- 1 cup cherry tomatoes, diced
- 1/2 cup shredded cheddar cheese
- 1/4 cup chopped fresh cilantro
- 1/4 cup sour cream
- 1 head iceberg or butter lettuce, leaves separated

Instructions:

1. Cook Ground Turkey:
   - In a large skillet over medium heat, cook the ground turkey until browned. Drain excess fat if needed.

2. Prepare Bacon:

- Cook the bacon until crispy, then crumble it into small pieces.

3. Saute Onion and Garlic:
   - In the same skillet, heat olive oil and sauté chopped onion and minced garlic until softened.

4. Season Turkey Mixture:
   - Add the ground cumin, chili powder, salt, and pepper to the turkey mixture. Stir well to combine.

5. Combine Ingredients:
   - In a large bowl, combine the cooked turkey mixture, crumbled bacon, diced cherry tomatoes, shredded cheddar cheese, and chopped cilantro. Mix well.

6. Assemble Lettuce Cups:
   - Spoon the turkey and bacon mixture into the individual lettuce leaves, creating lettuce cups.

7. Garnish and Serve:
   - Garnish each cup with a dollop of sour cream. Serve the Turkey and Bacon Lettuce Cups immediately.

Nutritional Information (per serving - 2 lettuce cups):

- Calories: 350 kcal
- Protein: 25g
- Fat: 22g
- Carbohydrates: 10g

- Fiber: 3g

Note: Nutritional information is approximate and may vary based on specific ingredients used.

Mushroom and Spinach Stuffed Chicken

Prep Time: 20 minutes
Cook Time: 25 minutes
Total Time: 45 minutes
Servings: 4

Ingredients:

For Stuffed Chicken:

- 4 boneless, skinless chicken breasts
- Salt and pepper to taste
- 1 tablespoon olive oil

For Mushroom and Spinach Filling:

- 2 cups mushrooms, finely chopped
- 2 cups fresh spinach, chopped
- 1 small onion, finely chopped
- 2 cloves garlic, minced
- 1/2 cup feta cheese, crumbled
- 1/4 cup grated Parmesan cheese
- 1 teaspoon dried oregano
- Salt and pepper to taste

For Coating:

- 2 tablespoons melted butter
- 1 teaspoon garlic powder
- 1 teaspoon dried thyme

Instructions:

Mushroom and Spinach Filling:

1. Saute Vegetables:
   - In a skillet, heat olive oil over medium heat. Add chopped mushrooms, onion, and garlic. Saute until the vegetables are tender.

2. Add Spinach:
   - Add chopped spinach to the skillet and cook until wilted. Remove from heat.

3. Mix Cheese and Seasoning:
   - In a bowl, combine the sautéed vegetables with crumbled feta cheese, grated Parmesan cheese, dried oregano, salt, and pepper. Mix well.

Stuffed Chicken:

1. Preheat Oven:
   - Preheat the oven to 400°F (200°C).

2. Prepare Chicken Breasts:
   - Lay the chicken breasts flat and cut a pocket into each one, being careful not to cut through the other side.

3. Season Chicken:
   - Season the inside of each chicken breast with salt and pepper.

4. Stuff Chicken:

- Stuff each chicken breast with the mushroom and spinach filling.

5. Secure with Toothpicks:
   - Use toothpicks to secure the edges of the chicken breasts and keep the filling in place.

 Coating and Baking:

1. Mix Coating:
   - In a small bowl, mix melted butter with garlic powder and dried thyme.

2. Brush Chicken:
   - Brush the outside of each stuffed chicken breast with the butter mixture.

3. Bake:
   - Place the stuffed chicken breasts on a baking sheet and bake in the preheated oven for 25 minutes or until the chicken is cooked through.

4. Serve:
   - Remove toothpicks before serving. Serve the Mushroom and Spinach Stuffed Chicken warm.

 Nutritional Information (per serving):

- Calories: 350 kcal
- Protein: 35g
- Fat: 18g
- Carbohydrates: 8g
- Fiber: 3g

Note: Nutritional information is approximate and may vary based on specific ingredients used.

Egg Salad Cucumber Boats

Prep Time: 15 minutes
Total Time: 15 minutes
Servings: 4

Ingredients:

- 4 large cucumbers
- 6 hard-boiled eggs, chopped
- 1/4 cup mayonnaise
- 1 tablespoon Dijon mustard
- 2 green onions, finely chopped
- 1 celery stalk, finely chopped
- 1 tablespoon fresh dill, chopped
- Salt and pepper to taste
- Paprika for garnish (optional)

Instructions:

1. Prepare Cucumbers:
    - Wash the cucumbers and cut them in half lengthwise. Using a spoon, scoop out the seeds to create a hollow center, forming cucumber boats.

2. Make Egg Salad:
    - In a bowl, combine chopped hard-boiled eggs, mayonnaise, Dijon mustard, green onions, celery, and fresh dill. Mix well.

3. Season Egg Salad:

- Season the egg salad with salt and pepper to taste. Adjust the seasoning as needed.

4. Fill Cucumber Boats:
   - Spoon the egg salad mixture into the hollowed-out center of each cucumber boat.

5. Garnish:
   - Garnish the Egg Salad Cucumber Boats with a sprinkle of paprika for added color and flavor (optional).

6. Serve:
   - Arrange the cucumber boats on a serving platter and serve immediately.

Nutritional Information (per serving - 1 cucumber boat):

- Calories: 180 kcal
- Protein: 10g
- Fat: 14g
- Carbohydrates: 5g
- Fiber: 2g

Note: Nutritional information is approximate and may vary based on specific ingredients used.

Shrimp and Zucchini Noodles

Prep Time: 20 minutes
Cook Time: 10 minutes
Total Time: 30 minutes
Servings: 4

Ingredients:

- 1lb large shrimp, peeled and deveined
- 4 medium zucchinis, spiralized into noodles
- 2 tablespoons olive oil
- 4 cloves garlic, minced
- 1 teaspoon red pepper flakes (optional)
- Salt and black pepper to taste
- Juice of 1 lemon
- 1/4 cup chopped fresh parsley
- Grated Parmesan cheese for garnish (optional)

Instructions:

1. Prepare Shrimp:
   - In a large skillet, heat 1 tablespoon of olive oil over medium-high heat. Add the shrimp and cook for 2-3 minutes per side or until they turn pink and opaque. Remove the shrimp from the skillet and set aside.

2. Saute Garlic and Red Pepper Flakes:
   - In the same skillet, add the remaining tablespoon of olive oil. Add minced garlic and red

pepper flakes (if using) and sauté for 1-2 minutes until fragrant.

3. Cook Zucchini Noodles:
   - Add the spiralized zucchini noodles to the skillet. Toss and cook for 2-3 minutes until they are just tender but still have a slight crunch.

4. Combine Shrimp and Zucchini:
   - Return the cooked shrimp to the skillet with the zucchini noodles. Toss everything together until well combined.

5. Season and Finish:
   - Season with salt and black pepper to taste. Squeeze the lemon juice over the shrimp and zucchini noodles. Toss again to evenly distribute the flavors.

6. Garnish and Serve:
   - Garnish with chopped fresh parsley and, if desired, grated Parmesan cheese. Serve the Shrimp and Zucchini Noodles immediately.

Nutritional Information (per serving):

- Calories: 220 kcal
- Protein: 25g
- Fat: 10g
- Carbohydrates: 10g
- Fiber: 3g

Note: Nutritional information is approximate and may vary based on specific ingredients used.

Cauliflower Fried Rice with Chicken

Prep Time: 20 minutes
Cook Time: 15 minutes
Total Time: 35 minutes
Servings: 4

Ingredients:

- 1 head cauliflower, riced (about 4 cups)
- 1lb boneless, skinless chicken breasts, diced
- 2 tablespoons sesame oil
- 4 cloves garlic, minced
- 1 tablespoon ginger, grated
- 1 cup carrots, diced
- 1 cup peas (fresh or frozen)
- 2 eggs, beaten
- 1/4 cup low-sodium soy sauce
- 2 green onions, sliced
- Salt and pepper to taste
- Sesame seeds for garnish (optional)

Instructions:

1. Prepare Cauliflower Rice:
   - Cut the cauliflower into florets and pulse in a food processor until it resembles rice. Set aside.

2. Cook Chicken:
   - In a large skillet or wok, heat 1 tablespoon of sesame oil over medium-high heat. Add diced chicken and cook until browned and cooked

through. Remove chicken from the skillet and set aside.

3. Saute Aromatics:
   - In the same skillet, add the remaining tablespoon of sesame oil. Add minced garlic and grated ginger, sautéing for 1-2 minutes until fragrant.

4. Cook Vegetables:
   - Add diced carrots and peas to the skillet. Stir-fry for 3-4 minutes until the vegetables are tender-crisp.

5. Add Cauliflower Rice:
   - Add the riced cauliflower to the skillet, stirring to combine with the vegetables.

6. Create Well in the Center:
   - Push the cauliflower mixture to the edges of the skillet, creating a well in the center.

7. Scramble Eggs:
   - Pour the beaten eggs into the well. Allow them to set slightly before stirring to scramble and mix with the cauliflower mixture.

8. Combine Chicken:
   - Return the cooked chicken to the skillet, tossing everything together.

9. Season with Soy Sauce:

- Pour the low-sodium soy sauce over the cauliflower fried rice. Stir well to evenly distribute the flavors. Season with salt and pepper to taste.

10. Garnish and Serve:
    - Garnish with sliced green onions and sesame seeds if desired. Serve the Cauliflower Fried Rice with Chicken hot.

Nutritional Information (per serving):

- Calories: 280 kcal
- Protein: 30g
- Fat: 10g
- Carbohydrates: 20g
- Fiber: 8g

Note: Nutritional information is approximate and may vary based on specific ingredients used.

Tuna Salad Stuffed Bell Peppers

Prep Time: 15 minutes
Total Time: 15 minutes
Servings: 4

Ingredients:

- 4 large bell peppers, halved and seeds removed
- 2 cans (5 oz each) tuna, drained
- 1/2 cup mayonnaise
- 1 celery stalk, finely chopped
- 1/4 cup red onion, finely chopped
- 2 tablespoons dill pickles, finely chopped
- 1 tablespoon Dijon mustard
- Salt and pepper to taste
- 1/4 cup fresh parsley, chopped, for garnish
- Lemon wedges for serving (optional)

Instructions:

1. Prepare Bell Peppers:
   - Cut the bell peppers in half, removing the seeds and membranes. Rinse them and set aside.

2. Make Tuna Salad:
   - In a bowl, combine drained tuna, mayonnaise, chopped celery, red onion, dill pickles, Dijon mustard, salt, and pepper. Mix well until all ingredients are evenly combined.

3. Stuff Bell Peppers:

- Spoon the tuna salad mixture into each bell pepper half, filling them evenly.

4. Garnish:
- Garnish the Tuna Salad Stuffed Bell Peppers with chopped fresh parsley.

5. Serve:
- Serve the stuffed bell peppers chilled. Optionally, serve with lemon wedges on the side for a burst of citrus flavor.

Nutritional Information (per serving - 1 stuffed bell pepper half):

- Calories: 220 kcal
- Protein: 15g
- Fat: 15g
- Carbohydrates: 5g
- Fiber: 2g

Note: Nutritional information is approximate and may vary based on specific ingredients used.

Caprese Zoodle Salad

Prep Time: 15 minutes
Total Time: 15 minutes
Servings: 4

Ingredients:

- 4 medium zucchinis, spiralized into noodles
- 1-pint cherry tomatoes, halved
- 8 oz fresh mozzarella, diced
- 1/4 cup fresh basil leaves, torn
- 2 tablespoons extra-virgin olive oil
- 1 tablespoon balsamic vinegar
- Salt and pepper to taste
- Balsamic glaze for drizzling (optional)
- Pine nuts for garnish (optional)

Instructions:

1. Prepare Zoodles:
    - Spiralize the zucchinis into noodles using a spiralizer. Place the zoodles in a large salad bowl.

2. Add Cherry Tomatoes:
    - Halve the cherry tomatoes and add them to the bowl with the zoodles.

3. Combine Mozzarella and Basil:
    - Dice the fresh mozzarella and tear the basil leaves. Add them to the bowl.

4. Dress the Salad:
   - In a small bowl, whisk together extra-virgin olive oil, balsamic vinegar, salt, and pepper. Drizzle the dressing over the zoodle mixture.

5. Toss and Coat:
   - Gently toss the ingredients until the zoodles are coated evenly with the dressing.

6. Garnish and Serve:
   - Optionally, drizzle with balsamic glaze and sprinkle with pine nuts for added flavor and crunch. Serve the Caprese Zoodle Salad immediately.

 Nutritional Information (per serving):

- Calories: 180 kcal
- Protein: 10g
- Fat: 14g
- Carbohydrates: 10g
- Fiber: 3g

Note: Nutritional information is approximate and may vary based on specific ingredients used.

Pesto Chicken Salad Lettuce Wraps

Prep Time: 20 minutes
Total Time: 20 minutes
Servings: 4

Ingredients:

For Pesto Chicken Salad:

- 2 cups cooked chicken breast, shredded
- 1/4 cup pesto sauce (store-bought or homemade)
- 1/4 cup mayonnaise
- 2 tablespoons pine nuts, toasted
- 1/4 cup sun-dried tomatoes, chopped
- Salt and pepper to taste

For Lettuce Wraps:

- 1 head iceberg or butter lettuce, leaves separated
- 1 cup cherry tomatoes, halved
- 1/2 cucumber, thinly sliced
- 1/4 cup red onion, thinly sliced
- Fresh basil leaves for garnish

Instructions:

Pesto Chicken Salad:

1. Prepare Chicken:
   - Cook and shred the chicken breasts. Allow them to cool.

2. Make Pesto Chicken Salad:
   - In a bowl, combine shredded chicken, pesto sauce, mayonnaise, toasted pine nuts, and chopped sun-dried tomatoes. Mix well. Season with salt and pepper to taste.

 Lettuce Wraps:

1. Prepare Lettuce Leaves:
   - Wash and separate the leaves of iceberg or butter lettuce.

2. Assemble Wraps:
  - On each lettuce leaf, spoon a generous portion of the pesto chicken salad.

3. Add Fresh Vegetables:
   - Top the chicken salad with halved cherry tomatoes, thinly sliced cucumber, and red onion.

4. Garnish:
  - Garnish each wrap with fresh basil leaves.

5. Serve:
   - Serve the Pesto Chicken Salad Lettuce Wraps immediately.

 Nutritional Information (per serving - 2 lettuce wraps):

- Calories: 280 kcal
- Protein: 25g

- Fat: 18g
- Carbohydrates: 10g
- Fiber: 3g

Note: Nutritional information is approximate and may vary based on specific ingredients used.

Beef and Broccoli Stir-Fry

Prep Time: 20 minutes
Cook Time: 10 minutes
Total Time: 30 minutes
Servings: 4

Ingredients:

For Beef Marinade:

- 1 lb flank steak, thinly sliced
- 2 tablespoons soy sauce
- 1 tablespoon oyster sauce
- 1 tablespoon cornstarch
- 1 teaspoon sesame oil
- 1 teaspoon sugar
- 1/2 teaspoon black pepper

For Stir-Fry:

- 2 tablespoons vegetable oil
- 3 cups broccoli florets
- 3 cloves garlic, minced
- 1 tablespoon ginger, grated
- 1/4 cup soy sauce
- 2 tablespoons oyster sauce
- 1 tablespoon hoisin sauce
- 1 tablespoon cornstarch mixed with 2 tablespoons
water (slurry)

Optional Garnish:

- Sesame seeds
- Sliced green onions

Instructions:

Beef Marinade:

1. Slice Beef:
   - Thinly slice the flank steak against the grain.

2. Marinate Beef:
   - In a bowl, combine sliced beef with soy sauce, oyster sauce, cornstarch, sesame oil, sugar, and black pepper. Mix well and let it marinate for at least 15 minutes.

Stir-Fry:

1. Prepare Broccoli:
   - Blanch or steam broccoli florets until slightly tender. Set aside.

2. Heat Oil:
   - In a wok or large skillet, heat vegetable oil over high heat.

3. Cook Beef:
   - Add marinated beef to the hot oil. Stir-fry for 2-3 minutes or until the beef is browned and cooked through. Remove beef from the wok and set aside.

4. Sauté Aromatics:

- In the same wok, add minced garlic and grated ginger. Sauté for 1-2 minutes until fragrant.

5. Add Broccoli:
   - Add the blanched broccoli to the wok. Stir-fry for another 2 minutes.

6. Combine Sauces:
   - In a small bowl, mix soy sauce, oyster sauce, and hoisin sauce. Pour the sauce mixture into the wok.

7. Thicken Sauce:
   - Pour the cornstarch slurry into the wok, stirring constantly. Allow the sauce to thicken.

8. Add Beef:
   - Return the cooked beef to the wok. Toss everything together until well-coated in the sauce.

9. Garnish and Serve:
   - Garnish with sesame seeds and sliced green onions if desired. Serve the Beef and Broccoli Stir-Fry over rice or noodles.

Nutritional Information (per serving):

- Calories: 350 kcal
- Protein: 25g
- Fat: 18g
- Carbohydrates: 20g
- Fiber: 4g

Note: Nutritional information is approximate and may vary based on specific ingredients used.

Cobb Salad with Ranch Dressing

Prep Time: 20 minutes
Total Time: 20 minutes
Servings: 4

Ingredients:

For Salad:

- 6 cups mixed salad greens (lettuce, spinach, arugula, etc.)
- 1 lb cooked chicken breast, diced
- 8 slices bacon, cooked and crumbled
- 4 large eggs, hard-boiled and chopped
- 1 cup cherry tomatoes, halved
- 1 avocado, diced
- 1/2 cup blue cheese, crumbled

For Ranch Dressing:

- 1/2 cup mayonnaise
- 1/2 cup buttermilk
- 1/4 cup sour cream
- 2 tablespoons fresh parsley, chopped
- 1 tablespoon fresh chives, chopped
- 1 teaspoon Dijon mustard
- 1 clove garlic, minced
- Salt and pepper to taste

Instructions:

Ranch Dressing:

1. Prepare Dressing:
   - In a bowl, whisk together mayonnaise, buttermilk, sour cream, chopped parsley, chopped chives, Dijon mustard, minced garlic, salt, and pepper. Refrigerate until ready to use.

 Salad:

1. Assemble Salad:
   - On a large serving platter or individual plates, arrange the mixed salad greens.

2. Arrange Ingredients:
   - Arrange diced chicken, crumbled bacon, chopped hard-boiled eggs, cherry tomatoes, diced avocado, and crumbled blue cheese in separate sections over the salad greens.

3. Serve with Ranch Dressing:
   - Drizzle the Cobb Salad with Ranch Dressing or serve the dressing on the side.

Nutritional Information (per serving):

- Calories: 480 kcal
- Protein: 30g
- Fat: 36g
- Carbohydrates: 15g
- Fiber: 6g

Note: Nutritional information is approximate and may vary based on specific ingredients used.

Eggplant Lasagna

Prep Time: 30 minutes
Cook Time: 45 minutes
Total Time: 1 hour 15 minutes
Servings: 6

Ingredients:

For Eggplant Layers:

- 2 large eggplants, thinly sliced lengthwise
- 2 tablespoons olive oil
- Salt and pepper to taste

For Meat Sauce:

- 1lb ground beef or turkey
- 1 onion, finely chopped
- 3 cloves garlic, minced
- 1 can (14 oz) crushed tomatoes
- 1 can (6 oz) tomato paste
- 1 teaspoon dried oregano
- 1 teaspoon dried basil
- Salt and pepper to taste

For Cheese Filling:

- 2 cups ricotta cheese
- 1 cup mozzarella cheese, shredded
- 1/2 cup Parmesan cheese, grated
- 1 egg

- 2 tablespoons fresh parsley, chopped
- Salt and pepper to taste

 Additional Layers:

- 2 cups mozzarella cheese, shredded

Instructions:

 Eggplant Layers:

1. Preheat Oven:
   - Preheat the oven to 375°F (190°C).

2. Slice Eggplant:
   - Slice the eggplants lengthwise into thin slices.

3. Season Eggplant:
   - Brush the eggplant slices with olive oil and season with salt and pepper. Bake in the preheated oven for 15-20 minutes or until tender.

 Meat Sauce:

1. Cook Meat:
   - In a skillet, cook the ground beef or turkey over medium heat until browned. Drain excess fat.

2. Add Aromatics:
   - Add chopped onion and minced garlic to the skillet. Sauté until the onion is translucent.

3. Combine Ingredients:
   - Stir in crushed tomatoes, tomato paste, dried oregano, dried basil, salt, and pepper. Simmer for 10-15 minutes.

Cheese Filling:

1. Prepare Cheese Mixture:
   - In a bowl, combine ricotta cheese, shredded mozzarella, Parmesan cheese, egg, chopped parsley, salt, and pepper.

Assemble Lasagna:

1. Layer Eggplant and Sauce:
   - In a greased baking dish, layer half of the baked eggplant slices. Top with half of the meat sauce.

2. Add Cheese Filling:
   - Spoon half of the cheese mixture over the meat sauce layer.

3. Repeat Layers:
   - Repeat the layers with the remaining eggplant, meat sauce, and cheese mixture.

4. Top with Mozzarella:
   - Sprinkle shredded mozzarella cheese over the top.

5. Bake:

- Cover the baking dish with foil and bake in the preheated oven for 30 minutes. Remove the foil and bake for an additional 15 minutes or until the cheese is bubbly and golden.

6. Rest and Serve:
   - Allow the Eggplant Lasagna to rest for 10 minutes before serving.

Nutritional Information (per serving):

- Calories: 420 kcal
- Protein: 28g
- Fat: 28g
- Carbohydrates: 16g
- Fiber: 7g

Note: Nutritional information is approximate and may vary based on specific ingredients used.

Avocado Tuna Boats

Prep Time: 15 minutes
Total Time: 15 minutes
Servings: 4

Ingredients:

- 4 large avocados, halved and pitted
- 2 cans (5 oz each) tuna, drained
- 1/2 cup red onion, finely chopped
- 1/2 cup celery, finely chopped
- 1/4 cup mayonnaise
- 1 tablespoon Dijon mustard
- 1 tablespoon fresh lemon juice
- Salt and pepper to taste
- Fresh parsley, chopped, for garnish

Instructions:

1. Prepare Avocado Halves:
   - Cut the avocados in half and remove the pits. Scoop out a small portion of the flesh to create a well for the tuna filling.

2. Make Tuna Salad:
   - In a bowl, combine drained tuna, chopped red onion, chopped celery, mayonnaise, Dijon mustard, and fresh lemon juice. Mix well. Season with salt and pepper to taste.

3. Fill Avocado Boats:

- Spoon the tuna salad mixture into the well of each avocado half.

4. Garnish:
   - Garnish the Avocado Tuna Boats with chopped fresh parsley.

5. Serve:
   - Serve immediately and enjoy these delicious and nutritious Avocado Tuna Boats.

Nutritional Information (per serving - 1 avocado boat):

- Calories: 320 kcal
- Protein: 20g
- Fat: 25g
- Carbohydrates: 10g
- Fiber: 7g

Note: Nutritional information is approximate and may vary based on specific ingredients used.

Spinach and Feta Stuffed Bell Peppers

Prep Time: 20 minutes
Cook Time: 25 minutes
Total Time: 45 minutes
Servings: 4

Ingredients:

- 4 large bell peppers, halved and seeds removed
- 2 tablespoons olive oil
- 1 onion, finely chopped
- 2 cloves garlic, minced
- 6 cups fresh spinach, chopped
- 1 cup feta cheese, crumbled
- 1 cup cooked quinoa or rice
- 1 teaspoon dried oregano
- Salt and pepper to taste
- 1 cup tomato sauce (for topping)
- Fresh parsley, chopped, for garnish

Instructions:

1. Preheat Oven:
   - Preheat the oven to 375°F (190°C).

2. Prepare Bell Peppers:
   - Cut the bell peppers in half, removing the seeds
and membranes. Rinse them and set aside.

3. Saute Spinach Mixture:

    - In a large skillet, heat olive oil over medium heat. Add chopped onion and minced garlic. Cook until the onion is translucent.

4. Add Spinach:
    - Add chopped spinach to the skillet and sauté until wilted.

5. Combine Ingredients:
    - In a large bowl, combine the sautéed spinach mixture, crumbled feta cheese, cooked quinoa or rice, dried oregano, salt, and pepper. Mix well.

6. Stuff Bell Peppers:
    - Spoon the spinach and feta mixture into each bell pepper half, pressing down gently.

7. Top with Tomato Sauce:
  - Pour tomato sauce over the stuffed bell peppers.

8. Bake:
  - Place the stuffed bell peppers in a baking dish. Cover with foil and bake in the preheated oven for 20 minutes. Uncover and bake for an additional 5 minutes or until the peppers are tender.

9. Garnish and Serve:
    - Garnish with chopped fresh parsley before serving.

 Nutritional Information (per serving - 1 stuffed bell pepper half):

- Calories: 280 kcal
- Protein: 12g
- Fat: 14g
- Carbohydrates: 28g
- Fiber: 6g

Note: Nutritional information is approximate and may vary based on specific ingredients used.

Cajun Shrimp and Sausage Skillet

Prep Time: 15 minutes
Cook Time: 20 minutes
Total Time: 35 minutes
Servings: 4

Ingredients:

- 1lb large shrimp, peeled and deveined
- 12 oz Andouille sausage, sliced
- 1 tablespoon olive oil
- 1 onion, diced
- 1 bell pepper, diced
- 3 cloves garlic, minced
- 1 can (14 oz) diced tomatoes, undrained
- 1 cup chicken broth
- 2 teaspoons Cajun seasoning
- 1 teaspoon dried thyme
- 1 teaspoon paprika
- 1/2 teaspoon cayenne pepper (adjust to taste)
- Salt and black pepper to taste
- Fresh parsley, chopped, for garnish
- Cooked rice or cauliflower rice, for serving

Instructions:

1. Prepare Shrimp and Sausage:
    - Pat the shrimp dry and season with Cajun seasoning. Set aside. Slice the Andouille sausage.

2. Sauté Sausage and Shrimp:

   - In a large skillet, heat olive oil over medium-high heat. Add sliced sausage and cook until browned. Add shrimp and cook until they turn pink. Remove sausage and shrimp from the skillet and set aside.

3. Sauté Vegetables:
   - In the same skillet, add diced onion, bell pepper, and minced garlic. Sauté until the vegetables are softened.

4. Combine **Ingredients:**
   - Pour in diced tomatoes with their juice. Add chicken broth, dried thyme, paprika, cayenne pepper, salt, and black pepper. Stir to combine.

5. Simmer:
   - Allow the mixture to simmer for 10 minutes, letting the flavors meld.

6. Add Sausage and Shrimp:
   - Return the cooked sausage and shrimp to the skillet. Stir to combine and let it simmer for an additional 5 minutes.

7. Adjust Seasoning:
   - Taste and adjust the seasoning if needed. If you prefer more heat, add extra Cajun seasoning or cayenne pepper.

8. Garnish and Serve:

- Garnish with chopped fresh parsley. Serve the Cajun Shrimp and Sausage over cooked rice or cauliflower rice.

Nutritional Information (per serving):

- Calories: 380 kcal
- Protein: 28g
- Fat: 22g
- Carbohydrates: 20g
- Fiber: 4g

Note: Nutritional information is approximate and may vary based on specific ingredients used.

Broccoli and Cheddar Soup

Prep Time: 15 minutes
Cook Time: 25 minutes
Total Time: 40 minutes
Servings: 6

Ingredients:

- 1/4 cup unsalted butter
- 1 onion, chopped
- 2 cloves garlic, minced
- 1/4 cup all-purpose flour
- 4 cups chicken or vegetable broth
- 4 cups fresh broccoli florets
- 1 carrot, grated
- 2 cups sharp cheddar cheese, shredded
- 1 cup whole milk or half-and-half
- Salt and pepper to taste
- Pinch of nutmeg (optional)
- Croutons or additional shredded cheddar for garnish (optional)

Instructions:

1. Sauté Vegetables:
   - In a large pot, melt butter over medium heat. Add chopped onion and garlic, sauté until softened.

2. Make Roux:
   - Stir in flour to create a roux. Cook for 2-3 minutes, stirring constantly.

3. Add Broth:
   - Gradually whisk in the chicken or vegetable broth to avoid lumps. Bring to a simmer.

4. Add Broccoli and Carrot:
   - Add broccoli florets and grated carrot to the pot. Simmer for 15-20 minutes or until vegetables are tender.

5. Blend Soup:
   - Use an immersion blender to blend the soup until smooth. Alternatively, transfer a portion of the soup to a blender, blend, and return to the pot.

6. Add Cheese and Milk:
   - Stir in shredded cheddar cheese until melted. Pour in whole milk or half-and-half, stirring continuously. Add salt, pepper, and a pinch of nutmeg if desired.

7. Adjust Consistency:
   - If the soup is too thick, add more broth or milk to reach your desired consistency.

8. Simmer and Serve:
   - Simmer the soup for an additional 5 minutes to meld the flavors. Adjust seasoning as needed.

9. Garnish and Serve:
   - Ladle the Broccoli and Cheddar Soup into bowls. Garnish with croutons or additional shredded cheddar if desired.

Nutritional Information (per serving):

- Calories: 350 kcal
- Protein: 16g
- Fat: 26g
- Carbohydrates: 18g
- Fiber: 4g

Note: Nutritional information is approximate and may vary based on specific ingredients used.

Greek Chicken Salad

Prep Time: 20 minutes
Cook Time: 15 minutes (for chicken)
Total Time: 35 minutes
Servings: 4

Ingredients:

For Grilled Chicken:

- 1lb boneless, skinless chicken breasts
- 2 tablespoons olive oil
- 1 teaspoon dried oregano
- 1 teaspoon garlic powder
- Salt and black pepper to taste

For Salad:

- 6 cups mixed salad greens (lettuce, spinach, arugula)
- 1 cucumber, sliced
- 1 cup cherry tomatoes, halved
- 1/2 red onion, thinly sliced
- 1/2 cup Kalamata olives, pitted
- 1/2 cup crumbled feta cheese
- Fresh parsley, chopped, for garnish

For Greek Salad Dressing:

- 1/4 cup extra-virgin olive oil
- 2 tablespoons red wine vinegar

- 1 teaspoon Dijon mustard
- 1 teaspoon dried oregano
- 1 clove garlic, minced
- Salt and black pepper to taste

Instructions:

Grilled Chicken:

1. Preheat Grill or Pan:
   - Preheat a grill or grill pan over medium-high heat.

2. Season Chicken:
   - In a bowl, mix olive oil, dried oregano, garlic powder, salt, and black pepper. Coat the chicken breasts with the mixture.

3. Grill Chicken:
   - Grill the chicken for about 6-7 minutes per side or until fully cooked. Allow it to rest for a few minutes before slicing.

Greek Salad:

1. Prepare Vegetables:
   - In a large salad bowl, combine mixed greens, sliced cucumber, halved cherry tomatoes, thinly sliced red onion, Kalamata olives, and crumbled feta cheese.

2. Add Grilled Chicken:

   - Slice the grilled chicken and arrange it over the salad.

 Greek Salad Dressing:

1. Prepare Dressing:
  - In a small bowl, whisk together extra-virgin olive oil, red wine vinegar, Dijon mustard, dried oregano, minced garlic, salt, and black pepper.

2. Dress Salad:
  - Drizzle the Greek Salad Dressing over the salad and gently toss to coat.

3. Garnish and Serve:
  - Garnish with chopped fresh parsley. Serve the Greek Chicken Salad immediately.

 Nutritional Information (per serving):

- Calories: 380 kcal
- Protein: 28g
- Fat: 24g
- Carbohydrates: 18g
- Fiber: 5g

Note: Nutritional information is approximate and may vary based on specific ingredients used.

Zucchini and Chicken Enchiladas

Prep Time: 30 minutes
Cook Time: 25 minutes
Total Time: 55 minutes
Servings: 4

Ingredients:

For Filling:

- 1lb boneless, skinless chicken breasts, cooked and shredded
- 2 medium zucchinis, grated
- 1 cup black beans, drained and rinsed
- 1 cup corn kernels (fresh or frozen)
- 1 cup shredded Monterey Jack cheese
- 1 teaspoon ground cumin
- 1 teaspoon chili powder
- Salt and black pepper to taste
- 1/4 cup fresh cilantro, chopped

For Enchilada Sauce:

- 2 cups red enchilada sauce (store-bought or homemade)

For Assembly:

- 8 medium-sized flour or corn tortillas
- 1 cup shredded cheddar cheese (for topping)
- Fresh cilantro, chopped (for garnish)

- Sour cream and sliced jalapeños (optional, for serving)

Instructions:

Filling:

1. Preheat Oven:
   - Preheat the oven to 375°F (190°C).

2. Prepare Filling:
   - In a large bowl, combine shredded chicken, grated zucchini, black beans, corn, Monterey Jack cheese, ground cumin, chili powder, salt, black pepper, and chopped cilantro. Mix well.

Enchilada Sauce:

1. Warm Enchilada Sauce:
   - In a saucepan, heat the red enchilada sauce over low heat until warmed.

Assembly:

1. Warm Tortillas:
   - If using corn tortillas, warm them in a dry skillet for a few seconds on each side. If using flour tortillas, you can warm them in the microwave.

2. Fill and Roll:
   - Spoon the filling onto each tortilla, roll them up, and place them seam side down in a greased baking dish.

3. Top with Sauce and Cheese:
   - Pour the warm enchilada sauce over the rolled tortillas. Sprinkle shredded cheddar cheese on top.

4. Bake:
   - Bake in the preheated oven for 20-25 minutes or until the cheese is melted and bubbly.

5. Garnish and Serve:
   - Garnish with chopped fresh cilantro. Serve the Zucchini and Chicken Enchiladas with optional sour cream and sliced jalapeños.

Nutritional Information (per serving - 2 enchiladas):

- Calories: 480 kcal
- Protein: 35g
- Fat: 20g
- Carbohydrates: 45g
- Fiber: 8g

Note: Nutritional information is approximate and may vary based on specific ingredients used.

Mediterranean Quinoa Salad

Prep Time: 15 minutes
Cook Time: 15 minutes (for quinoa)
Total Time: 30 minutes

Servings: 6

Ingredients:

For Salad:

- 1 cup quinoa, rinsed
- 2 cups water
- 1 cup cherry tomatoes, halved
- 1 cucumber, diced
- 1/2 red onion, finely chopped
- 1/2 cup Kalamata olives, pitted and sliced
- 1/2 cup crumbled feta cheese
- 1/4 cup fresh parsley, chopped
- 1/4 cup fresh mint, chopped

For Dressing:

- 1/4 cup extra-virgin olive oil
- 2 tablespoons red wine vinegar
- 1 clove garlic, minced
- 1 teaspoon dried oregano
- Salt and black pepper to taste
- Juice of 1 lemon

Instructions:

Quinoa:

1. Cook Quinoa:
   - In a saucepan, combine rinsed quinoa and water.
Bring to a boil, then reduce heat, cover, and simmer

for 15 minutes or until the quinoa is cooked and water is absorbed. Fluff with a fork and let it cool.

Salad:

1. Prepare Vegetables:
   - In a large bowl, combine cooked quinoa, halved cherry tomatoes, diced cucumber, finely chopped red onion, sliced Kalamata olives, crumbled feta cheese, chopped fresh parsley, and chopped fresh mint.

Dressing:

1. Whisk Dressing:
   - In a small bowl, whisk together extra-virgin olive oil, red wine vinegar, minced garlic, dried oregano, salt, black pepper, and lemon juice.

2. Toss Salad:
   - Pour the dressing over the salad and toss until all ingredients are well coated.

3. Chill:
   - Refrigerate the Mediterranean Quinoa Salad for at least 30 minutes before serving to allow the flavors to meld.

Nutritional Information (per serving):

- Calories: 280 kcal
- Protein: 8g
- Fat: 16g

- Carbohydrates: 28g
- Fiber: 5g

Note: Nutritional information is approximate and may vary based on specific ingredients used.

Spaghetti Squash with Meatballs

Prep Time: 20 minutes
Cook Time: 1 hour
Total Time: 1 hour 20 minutes
Servings: 4

Ingredients:

For Spaghetti Squash:

- 2 medium spaghetti squash, halved and seeds removed
- 2 tablespoons olive oil
- Salt and black pepper to taste

For Meatballs:

- 1lb ground beef
- 1/2 cup breadcrumbs
- 1/4 cup grated Parmesan cheese
- 1/4 cup fresh parsley, chopped
- 1 egg
- 2 cloves garlic, minced
- 1 teaspoon dried oregano
- Salt and black pepper to taste

For Tomato Sauce:

- 2 cups tomato sauce (store-bought or homemade)
- 1 teaspoon dried basil
- 1 teaspoon dried thyme

- 1/2 teaspoon red pepper flakes (optional)

 For Garnish:

- Fresh basil or parsley, chopped
- Grated Parmesan cheese

 Instructions:

 Spaghetti Squash:

1. Preheat Oven:
   - Preheat the oven to 400°F (200°C).

2. Prepare Squash:
     - Drizzle olive oil over the cut sides of the spaghetti squash. Season with salt and black pepper. Place the halves, cut side down, on a baking sheet.

3. Roast Squash:
   - Roast in the preheated oven for 40-45 minutes or until the squash is fork-tender. Scrape the flesh with a fork to create "spaghetti."

 Meatballs:

1. Preheat Oven:
   - Reduce the oven temperature to 375°F (190°C).

2. Prepare Meatball Mixture:
   - In a bowl, combine ground beef, breadcrumbs, grated Parmesan cheese, chopped fresh parsley,

egg, minced garlic, dried oregano, salt, and black pepper. Mix until well combined.

3. Form Meatballs:
   - Shape the mixture into meatballs, about 1 inch in diameter, and place them on a baking sheet.

4. Bake Meatballs:
   - Bake in the preheated oven for 20-25 minutes or until the meatballs are cooked through and browned.

Tomato Sauce:

1. Prepare Sauce:
   - In a saucepan, heat tomato sauce over medium heat. Add dried basil, dried thyme, and red pepper flakes if using. Simmer for 10 minutes.

Assemble:

1. Serve:
   - Place a portion of roasted spaghetti squash on each plate, top with meatballs, and spoon tomato sauce over the dish.

2. Garnish:
   - Garnish with chopped fresh basil or parsley and grated Parmesan cheese.

Nutritional Information (per serving):

- Calories: 420 kcal

- Protein: 25g
- Fat: 22g
- Carbohydrates: 35g
- Fiber: 8g

Note: Nutritional information is approximate and may vary based on specific ingredients used.

Asparagus and Ham Stuffed Chicken

Prep Time: 25 minutes
Cook Time: 30 minutes
Total Time: 55 minutes
Servings: 4

Ingredients:

For Stuffed Chicken:

- 4 boneless, skinless chicken breasts
- 1 bunch asparagus, ends trimmed
- 4 slices ham
- 1 cup shredded Swiss cheese
- Salt and black pepper to taste
- 1 tablespoon olive oil

For Seasoning:

- 1 teaspoon garlic powder
- 1 teaspoon onion powder
- 1 teaspoon dried thyme
- 1/2 teaspoon paprika
- 1/2 teaspoon dried rosemary
- Salt and black pepper to taste

Instructions:

Stuffed Chicken:

1. Preheat Oven:

- Preheat the oven to 375°F (190°C).

2. Butterfly Chicken Breasts:
   - Butterfly each chicken breast by slicing horizontally, creating a pocket for the stuffing. Be careful not to cut through.

3. Season Chicken:
   - In a small bowl, mix garlic powder, onion powder, dried thyme, paprika, dried rosemary, salt, and black pepper. Season both sides of each chicken breast with the seasoning.

4. Layer Ham and Asparagus:
   - Place a slice of ham inside each chicken breast, followed by a few asparagus spears. Top with shredded Swiss cheese.

5. Fold and Secure:
   - Fold the chicken breast over the stuffing ingredients, creating a stuffed pocket. Secure with toothpicks if needed.

6. Season Outside:
   - Brush the outside of each stuffed chicken breast with olive oil and sprinkle with salt and black pepper.

Bake:

1. Bake Chicken:
   - Place the stuffed chicken breasts in a baking dish. Bake in the preheated oven for 25-30 minutes

or until the chicken is cooked through and the cheese is melted and bubbly.

2. Broil (Optional):
   - If you desire a golden-brown crust, you can broil the stuffed chicken for an additional 2-3 minutes, watching closely to prevent burning.

Serve:

1. Rest and Slice:
   - Allow the stuffed chicken to rest for a few minutes before slicing. Remove any toothpicks.

2. Serve:
   - Serve the Asparagus and Ham Stuffed Chicken slices on a plate, and optionally drizzle with pan juices.

Nutritional Information (per serving):

- Calories: 350 kcal
- Protein: 40g
- Fat: 15g
- Carbohydrates: 8g
- Fiber: 3g

Note: Nutritional information is approximate and may vary based on specific ingredients used.

Turkey and Avocado Lettuce Wrap

Prep Time: 15 minutes
Total Time: 15 minutes
Servings: 4 wraps

Ingredients:

- 1lb lean ground turkey
- 1 tablespoon olive oil
- 1 teaspoon ground cumin
- 1 teaspoon chili powder
- 1/2 teaspoon garlic powder
- Salt and black pepper to taste
- 4 large lettuce leaves (such as iceberg or butter lettuce)
- 1 avocado, sliced
- 1 cup cherry tomatoes, halved
- 1/2 cup red onion, finely diced
- 1/4 cup fresh cilantro, chopped
- Juice of 1 lime

Instructions:

1. Cook Ground Turkey:
   - In a skillet over medium heat, add olive oil and ground turkey. Cook until browned and cooked through, breaking it apart with a spoon as it cooks.

2. Season Turkey:
   - Sprinkle ground cumin, chili powder, garlic powder, salt, and black pepper over the cooked

turkey. Stir well to incorporate the seasonings. Cook for an additional 2-3 minutes.

3. Prepare Lettuce Wraps:
    - Lay out the large lettuce leaves on a clean surface.

4. Assemble Wraps:
    - Spoon the seasoned ground turkey onto each lettuce leaf.

5. Add Toppings:
    - Top the turkey with sliced avocado, halved cherry tomatoes, finely diced red onion, and chopped cilantro.

6. Drizzle Lime Juice:
    - Squeeze lime juice over each wrap for a burst of freshness.

7. Fold and Serve:
    - Carefully fold the sides of the lettuce leaves over the filling, creating a wrap. Secure with toothpicks if needed.

Nutritional Information (per wrap):

- Calories: 280 kcal
- Protein: 25g
- Fat: 15g
- Carbohydrates: 12g
- Fiber: 6g

Note: Nutritional information is approximate and may vary based on specific ingredients used.

Cabbage and Beef Stir-Fry

Prep Time: 15 minutes
Cook Time: 15 minutes
Total Time: 30 minutes
Servings: 4

Ingredients:

- 1lb lean ground beef
- 2 tablespoons vegetable oil
- 4 cups cabbage, thinly sliced
- 1 cup carrots, julienned
- 1 cup bell peppers (any color), thinly sliced
- 4 green onions, sliced
- 3 cloves garlic, minced
- 1 tablespoon fresh ginger, minced
- 1/4 cup low-sodium soy sauce
- 2 tablespoons oyster sauce
- 1 tablespoon sesame oil
- 1 tablespoon rice vinegar
- 1 teaspoon sugar
- 1/2 teaspoon red pepper flakes (optional)
- Salt and black pepper to taste
- Sesame seeds and chopped cilantro for garnish (optional)
- Cooked rice or cauliflower rice for serving

Instructions:

1. Prepare Ingredients:

- Thinly slice the cabbage, julienne the carrots, thinly slice the bell peppers, chop the green onions, mince the garlic, and grate the fresh ginger.

2. Cook Ground Beef:
   - In a large skillet or wok, heat vegetable oil over medium-high heat. Add the ground beef and cook until browned, breaking it apart with a spoon as it cooks.

3. Add Aromatics:
   - Add minced garlic and ginger to the cooked beef. Sauté for 1-2 minutes until fragrant.

4. Add Vegetables:
   - Add sliced cabbage, julienned carrots, sliced bell peppers, and green onions to the skillet. Stir-fry for 5-7 minutes or until the vegetables are tender-crisp.

5. Prepare Sauce:
   - In a small bowl, whisk together soy sauce, oyster sauce, sesame oil, rice vinegar, sugar, and red pepper flakes if using.

6. Sauce and Season:
   - Pour the sauce over the stir-fry and toss to coat. Season with salt and black pepper to taste. Cook for an additional 2-3 minutes.

7. Garnish and Serve:

- Garnish the stir-fry with sesame seeds and chopped cilantro if desired. Serve over cooked rice or cauliflower rice.

Nutritional Information (per serving):

- Calories: 350 kcal
- Protein: 25g
- Fat: 20g
- Carbohydrates: 18g
- Fiber: 6g

Note: Nutritional information is approximate and may vary based on specific ingredients used.

Creamy Avocado and Shrimp Salad

Prep Time: 15 minutes
Cook Time: 5 minutes
Total Time: 20 minutes
Servings: 4

Ingredients:

- 1 lb large shrimp, peeled and deveined
- 2 avocados, diced
- 1 cup cherry tomatoes, halved
- 1 cucumber, diced
- 1/4 cup red onion, finely chopped
- 1/4 cup fresh cilantro, chopped
- 2 tablespoons mayonnaise
- 2 tablespoons Greek yogurt
- 2 tablespoons lime juice
- 1 clove garlic, minced
- Salt and black pepper to taste
- Lettuce leaves for serving

Instructions:

1. Cook Shrimp:
   - In a pot of boiling water, cook the shrimp for 2-3 minutes or until they turn pink and opaque. Drain and let them cool.

2. Prepare Vegetables:

- Dice the avocados, halve the cherry tomatoes, dice the cucumber, finely chop the red onion, and chop the fresh cilantro.

3. Make Dressing:
   - In a small bowl, whisk together mayonnaise, Greek yogurt, lime juice, minced garlic, salt, and black pepper to create the creamy dressing.

4. Assemble Salad:
   - In a large bowl, combine the cooked shrimp, diced avocados, halved cherry tomatoes, diced cucumber, chopped red onion, and cilantro.

5. Add Dressing:
   - Pour the creamy dressing over the salad ingredients and gently toss to coat everything evenly.

6. Chill:
   - Refrigerate the salad for at least 15 minutes to let the flavors meld.

7. Serve:
   - Spoon the Creamy Avocado and Shrimp Salad onto individual lettuce leaves for a refreshing presentation.

Nutritional Information (per serving):

- Calories: 280 kcal
- Protein: 20g

- Fat: 18g
- Carbohydrates: 15g
- Fiber: 7g

Note: Nutritional information is approximate and may vary based on specific ingredients used.

Dinners

Grilled Lemon Garlic Chicken

Prep Time: 15 minutes
Marinating Time: 30 minutes to 4 hours
Cook Time: 15 minutes
Total Time: 1 hour (including marinating time)
Servings: 4

Ingredients:

- 4 boneless, skinless chicken breasts
- Zest and juice of 2 lemons
- 4 cloves garlic, minced
- 2 tablespoons olive oil
- 1 teaspoon dried oregano
- 1 teaspoon dried thyme
- 1 teaspoon paprika
- Salt and black pepper to taste
- Fresh parsley for garnish (optional)

Instructions:

1. Prepare Marinade:
    - In a bowl, combine lemon zest, lemon juice, minced garlic, olive oil, dried oregano, dried thyme, paprika, salt, and black pepper. Mix well to create the marinade.

2. Marinate Chicken:

- Place the chicken breasts in a resealable plastic bag or shallow dish. Pour the marinade over the chicken, ensuring each piece is coated. Seal the bag or cover the dish and refrigerate for at least 30 minutes, or up to 4 hours for more flavor.

3. Preheat Grill:
  - Preheat the grill to medium-high heat.

4. Grill Chicken:
   - Remove the chicken from the marinade and let any excess drip off. Grill the chicken breasts for about 6-8 minutes per side or until they reach an internal temperature of 165°F (74°C). Cooking times may vary based on the thickness of the chicken.

5. Rest and Garnish:
   - Remove the chicken from the grill and let it rest for a few minutes before slicing. Garnish with fresh parsley if desired.

6. Serve:
   - Serve the Grilled Lemon Garlic Chicken with your favorite side dishes, such as roasted vegetables, salad, or couscous.

Nutritional Information (per serving):

- Calories: 250 kcal

- Protein: 30g
- Fat: 10g
- Carbohydrates: 4g
- Fiber: 1g

Note: Nutritional information is approximate and may vary based on specific ingredients used.

Zucchini Noodles with Pesto Shrimp

Prep Time: 15 minutes
Cook Time: 10 minutes
Total Time: 25 minutes
Servings: 4

Ingredients:

For Pesto Shrimp:

- 1 lb large shrimp, peeled and deveined
- 2 tablespoons olive oil
- 1/2 cup fresh basil leaves
- 1/4 cup grated Parmesan cheese
- 2 cloves garlic, minced
- 1/4 cup pine nuts
- Juice of 1 lemon
- Salt and black pepper to taste

For Zucchini Noodles:

- 4 medium zucchinis, spiralized
- 2 tablespoons olive oil
- 2 cloves garlic, minced
- Salt and black pepper to taste
- Cherry tomatoes for garnish (optional)
- Grated Parmesan cheese for topping

Instructions:

Pesto Shrimp:

1. Prepare Pesto:
   - In a food processor, combine fresh basil, Parmesan cheese, minced garlic, pine nuts, lemon juice, salt, and black pepper. Pulse until well combined.

2. Cook Shrimp:
   - In a skillet over medium heat, heat olive oil. Add shrimp and cook for 2-3 minutes per side or until they turn pink and opaque.

3. Add Pesto:
   - Add the prepared pesto to the cooked shrimp in the skillet. Stir to coat the shrimp evenly. Cook for an additional 1-2 minutes until the flavors meld.

Zucchini Noodles:

1. Spiralize Zucchini:
   - Spiralize the zucchinis to create zucchini noodles.

2. Cook Zucchini Noodles:
   - In a separate skillet, heat olive oil over medium heat. Add minced garlic and cook for 1 minute. Add the zucchini noodles and toss for 2-3 minutes until they are just tender but still have a bit of crunch. Season with salt and black pepper.

3. Combine and Serve:

- Combine the pesto shrimp with the zucchini noodles. Toss gently to coat the noodles with the pesto.

4. Garnish:
   - Garnish with cherry tomatoes if desired and top with grated Parmesan cheese.

 Nutritional Information (per serving):

- Calories: 320 kcal
- Protein: 25g
- Fat: 20g
- Carbohydrates: 12g
- Fiber: 4g

Note: Nutritional information is approximate and may vary based on specific ingredients used.

Baked Cod with Herbed Butter

Prep Time: 15 minutes
Marinating Time: 30 minutes
Cook Time: 15 minutes
Total Time: 1 hour (including marinating time)
Servings: 4

Ingredients:

- 4 cod fillets
- 2 tablespoons olive oil
- 2 tablespoons fresh parsley, finely chopped
- 1 tablespoon fresh dill, chopped
- 1 tablespoon fresh chives, minced
- 2 cloves garlic, minced
- 1 lemon, zest and juice
- Salt and black pepper to taste
- Herbed butter for serving (optional)

Instructions:

1. Prepare Herbed Marinade:
   - In a bowl, combine olive oil, chopped parsley, chopped dill, minced chives, minced garlic, lemon zest, lemon juice, salt, and black pepper.

2. Marinate Cod:
   - Place the cod fillets in a shallow dish. Pour the herbed marinade over the fillets, ensuring they are well coated. Let it marinate in the refrigerator for at least 30 minutes.

3. Preheat Oven:
   - Preheat the oven to 375°F (190°C).

4. Bake Cod:
   - Transfer the marinated cod fillets to a baking dish. Bake for 15 minutes or until the fish flakes easily with a fork.

5. Serve:
   - Remove the baked cod from the oven. Serve it hot, drizzled with any remaining herbed marinade or a dollop of herbed butter if desired.

Nutritional Information (per serving):

- Calories: 180 kcal
- Protein: 25g
- Fat: 8g
- Carbohydrates: 2g
- Fiber: 1g

Note: Nutritional information is approximate and may vary based on specific ingredients used.

Stuffed Bell Peppers with Ground Turkey

Prep Time: 20 minutes
Cook Time: 40 minutes
Total Time: 1 hour
Servings: 4

Ingredients:

- 4 large bell peppers, halved and seeds removed
- 1lb lean ground turkey
- 1 cup cooked quinoa
- 1 cup black beans, drained and rinsed
- 1 cup corn kernels (fresh, frozen, or canned)
- 1 cup diced tomatoes
- 1/2 cup diced red onion
- 2 cloves garlic, minced
- 1 teaspoon ground cumin
- 1 teaspoon chili powder
- 1/2 teaspoon paprika
- Salt and black pepper to taste
- 1 cup shredded cheddar cheese
- Fresh cilantro for garnish (optional)
- Sour cream for serving (optional)

Instructions:

1. Preheat Oven:
   - Preheat the oven to 375°F (190°C).

2. Prepare Bell Peppers:

- Cut the bell peppers in half lengthwise and remove the seeds and membranes. Place the pepper halves in a baking dish.

3. Cook Ground Turkey:
   - In a skillet over medium heat, cook the ground turkey until browned. Drain any excess fat.

4. Combine Ingredients:
   - In a large mixing bowl, combine the cooked ground turkey, cooked quinoa, black beans, corn, diced tomatoes, diced red onion, minced garlic, ground cumin, chili powder, paprika, salt, and black pepper. Mix well.

5. Stuff Bell Peppers:
   - Spoon the turkey and quinoa mixture into each bell pepper half, pressing down gently.

6. Bake:
   - Top each stuffed pepper with shredded cheddar cheese. Cover the baking dish with foil and bake for 30 minutes. Remove the foil and bake for an additional 10 minutes or until the cheese is melted and bubbly.

7. Serve:
   - Garnish with fresh cilantro if desired. Serve the stuffed bell peppers hot, with a dollop of sour cream if you like.

Nutritional Information (per serving):

- Calories: 400 kcal
- Protein: 30g
- Fat: 10g
- Carbohydrates: 50g
- Fiber: 12g

Note: Nutritional information is approximate and may vary based on specific ingredients used.

Cauliflower Crust Pizza

Prep Time: 20 minutes
Cook Time: 25 minutes
Total Time: 45 minutes
Servings: 4

Ingredients:
For Cauliflower Crust:

- 1 medium-sized cauliflower head, riced (about 4 cups)
- 1/2 cup shredded mozzarella cheese
- 1/4 cup grated Parmesan cheese
- 1 teaspoon dried oregano
- 1 teaspoon garlic powder
- 1/2 teaspoon salt
- 1/4 teaspoon black pepper
- 2 large eggs

For Toppings:
- 1/2 cup pizza sauce
- 1 cup shredded mozzarella cheese
- Your favorite pizza toppings (e.g., sliced bell peppers, cherry tomatoes, olives, mushrooms, etc.)
- Fresh basil or parsley for garnish (optional)

Instructions:
For Cauliflower Crust:

1. Preheat Oven:
   - Preheat the oven to 400°F (200°C).

2. Prepare Cauliflower Rice:
   - Cut the cauliflower into florets and pulse in a food processor until it resembles rice.

3. Steam Cauliflower Rice:
   - Place the cauliflower rice in a microwave-safe bowl and microwave for 4-5 minutes or until softened. Alternatively, steam on the stovetop.

4. Drain and Cool:
   - Allow the steamed cauliflower rice to cool. Place it in a clean kitchen towel and squeeze out excess moisture.

5. Make Cauliflower Dough:
   - In a bowl, combine the cauliflower rice, shredded mozzarella, grated Parmesan, dried oregano, garlic powder, salt, black pepper, and eggs. Mix until well combined.

6. Shape the Crust:
   - Line a baking sheet with parchment paper. Spread the cauliflower mixture onto the parchment paper, shaping it into a round or rectangular crust.

7. Bake the Crust:
   - Bake for 15-18 minutes or until the crust is golden and holds together.

Assemble and Bake Pizza:

1. Preheat Oven:
   - Increase the oven temperature to 425°F (220°C).

2. Add Toppings:
   - Spread pizza sauce evenly over the cauliflower crust. Sprinkle with shredded mozzarella cheese and add your favorite toppings.

3. Bake Pizza:
   - Bake for an additional 10-12 minutes or until the cheese is melted and bubbly.

4. Garnish and Serve:
   - Garnish with fresh basil or parsley if desired. Slice and serve your delicious Cauliflower Crust Pizza.

Nutritional Information (per serving, without toppings):

- Calories: 180 kcal
- Protein: 12g
- Fat: 10g
- Carbohydrates: 14g
- Fiber: 6g

Note: Nutritional information is approximate and may vary based on specific ingredients used.

Spicy Beef Lettuce Wraps

Prep Time: 20 minutes
Cook Time: 15 minutes
Total Time: 35 minutes
Servings: 4

Ingredients:

For Spicy Beef Filling:

- 1lb lean ground beef
- 2 tablespoons soy sauce
- 1 tablespoon hoisin sauce
- 1 tablespoon oyster sauce
- 1 tablespoon Sriracha sauce (adjust to taste)
- 1 tablespoon vegetable oil
- 2 cloves garlic, minced
- 1 tablespoon ginger, minced
- 1/2 cup water chestnuts, finely chopped
- 1/4 cup green onions, sliced
- Salt and black pepper to taste

For Lettuce Wraps:

- 1 head iceberg or butter lettuce, leaves separated and washed
- 1 cup cooked jasmine rice (optional)
- Sesame seeds for garnish (optional)
- Extra sliced green onions for garnish (optional)

Instructions:

For Spicy Beef Filling:

1. Cook Ground Beef:
   - In a large skillet or wok, heat vegetable oil over medium-high heat. Add ground beef and cook until browned, breaking it apart with a spatula.

2. Add Aromatics:
   - Add minced garlic and ginger to the beef. Sauté for 1-2 minutes until fragrant.

3. Season the Beef:
   - Stir in soy sauce, hoisin sauce, oyster sauce, and Sriracha sauce. Mix well to coat the beef with the flavorful sauce.

4. Add Vegetables:
   - Add chopped water chestnuts and sliced green onions to the beef mixture. Cook for an additional 2-3 minutes.

5. Adjust Seasoning:
   - Taste and adjust the seasoning with salt and black pepper. If you prefer more heat, add extra Sriracha.

Assemble Lettuce Wraps:

1. Prepare Lettuce Leaves:
   - Wash and separate the leaves of iceberg or butter lettuce to create cups.

2. Fill Lettuce Cups:
   - Spoon the spicy beef mixture into each lettuce cup. If desired, add a spoonful of cooked jasmine rice to each cup.

3. Garnish:
   - Garnish the spicy beef with sesame seeds and extra sliced green onions.

4. Serve:
   - Serve the Spicy Beef Lettuce Wraps immediately. Encourage diners to pick up the wraps and enjoy the delicious combination of flavors.

Nutritional Information (per serving):

- Calories: 250 kcal
- Protein: 20g
- Fat: 14g
- Carbohydrates: 12g
- Fiber: 3g

Note: Nutritional information is approximate and may vary based on specific ingredients used.

Salmon and Broccoli Foil Packets

Prep Time: 15 minutes
Cook Time: 20 minutes
Total Time: 35 minutes
Servings: 4

Ingredients:

- 4 salmon fillets
- 4 cups broccoli florets
- 4 cloves garlic, minced
- 1 lemon, thinly sliced
- 2 tablespoons olive oil
- 1 teaspoon dried dill
- 1 teaspoon dried thyme
- Salt and black pepper to taste
- 4 tablespoons butter, divided
- Fresh dill for garnish (optional)
- Lemon wedges for serving

Instructions:

1. Preheat Oven:
   - Preheat the oven to 400°F (200°C).

2. Prepare Foil Packets:
   - Cut four pieces of aluminum foil, each large enough to wrap a salmon fillet and a portion of broccoli. Place a salmon fillet in the center of each foil piece.

3. Season Salmon:
   - Drizzle olive oil over each salmon fillet. Sprinkle minced garlic, dried dill, dried thyme, salt, and black pepper evenly over the fillets.

4. Add Broccoli:

   - Arrange broccoli florets around each salmon fillet. Place lemon slices on top of the salmon.

5. Dot with Butter:
   - Place a tablespoon of butter on top of each salmon fillet.

6. Wrap Foil Packets:
   - Fold the foil over the salmon and broccoli, sealing the edges to create a packet.

7. Bake:
   - Place the foil packets on a baking sheet and bake in the preheated oven for 18-20 minutes, or until the salmon is cooked through and flakes easily with a fork.

8. Serve:
   - Carefully open the foil packets, garnish with fresh dill if desired, and serve the Salmon and Broccoli Foil Packets hot. Accompany with lemon wedges for a burst of citrus flavor.

Nutritional Information (per serving):

- Calories: 350 kcal
- Protein: 30g
- Fat: 22g
- Carbohydrates: 12g
- Fiber: 4g

Note: Nutritional information is approximate and may vary based on specific ingredients used.

Eggplant Parmesan

Prep Time: 45 minutes
Cook Time: 30 minutes
Total Time: 1 hour 15 minutes
Servings: 4

Ingredients:

For Eggplant:

- 2 large eggplants, thinly sliced
- Salt for sweating eggplant
- 1 cup all-purpose flour
- 3 large eggs, beaten
- 2 cups breadcrumbs
- 1 cup grated Parmesan cheese
- Vegetable oil for frying

For Assembly:

- 2 cups marinara sauce
- 2 cups shredded mozzarella cheese
- 1/2 cup grated Parmesan cheese
- Fresh basil for garnish (optional)

Instructions:

For Eggplant:

1. Preheat Oven:
   - Preheat the oven to 375°F (190°C).

2. Sweat and Slice Eggplant:
   - Sprinkle eggplant slices with salt and let them sit for about 30 minutes to draw out moisture. Pat them dry with a paper towel.

3. Set Up Breading Station:
   - Set up a breading station with three shallow dishes: one with flour, one with beaten eggs, and one with a mixture of breadcrumbs and grated Parmesan.

4. Bread Eggplant Slices:
   - Dip each eggplant slice into the flour, then into the beaten eggs, and finally into the breadcrumb mixture, ensuring even coating.

5. Fry Eggplant:
   - In a large skillet, heat vegetable oil over medium-high heat. Fry the breaded eggplant slices until golden brown on both sides. Place them on a paper towel-lined plate to drain excess oil.

 For Assembly:

1. Layer Eggplant and Sauce:
   - In a baking dish, spread a thin layer of marinara sauce. Place a layer of fried eggplant slices on top.

2. Add Cheese:
   - Sprinkle shredded mozzarella and grated Parmesan over the eggplant layer.

3. Repeat Layers:
   - Repeat the layering process until all the eggplant is used, finishing with a generous layer of cheese on top.

4. Bake:
   - Bake in the preheated oven for 25-30 minutes or until the cheese is melted and bubbly.

5. Garnish and Serve:
   - Garnish with fresh basil if desired. Allow it to cool slightly before serving. Serve the Eggplant Parmesan hot.

Nutritional Information (per serving):

- Calories: 450 kcal
- Protein: 20g
- Fat: 25g
- Carbohydrates: 40g
- Fiber: 8g

Note: Nutritional information is approximate and may vary based on specific ingredients used.

Creamy Garlic Parmesan Chicken

Prep Time: 15 minutes
Cook Time: 20 minutes
Total Time: 35 minutes
Servings: 4

Ingredients:

- 4 boneless, skinless chicken breasts
- Salt and black pepper to taste
- 1 teaspoon garlic powder
- 1 teaspoon onion powder
- 1 teaspoon dried oregano
- 2 tablespoons olive oil
- 4 cloves garlic, minced
- 1 cup chicken broth
- 1 cup heavy cream
- 1 cup grated Parmesan cheese
- 1 cup spinach leaves
- Chopped fresh parsley for garnish (optional)

Instructions:

1. Season Chicken:
    - Season the chicken breasts with salt, black pepper, garlic powder, onion powder, and dried oregano on both sides.

2. Sear Chicken:
    - In a large skillet, heat olive oil over medium-high heat. Sear the chicken breasts for 4-5

minutes on each side until golden brown and cooked through. Remove the chicken from the skillet and set aside.

3. Make Creamy Garlic Parmesan Sauce:
   - In the same skillet, add minced garlic and sauté for 1-2 minutes until fragrant. Pour in the chicken broth, scraping any browned bits from the bottom of the pan.

4. Add Heavy Cream:
   - Add the heavy cream and bring the mixture to a simmer.

5. Melt Parmesan:
   - Stir in the grated Parmesan cheese and continue to simmer, stirring constantly, until the cheese is melted and the sauce is smooth.

6. Add Spinach:
   - Add spinach leaves to the sauce and let them wilt into the mixture.

7. Return Chicken:
   - Return the seared chicken breasts to the skillet, spooning some of the sauce over them.

8. Simmer:
   - Allow the chicken to simmer in the sauce for an additional 5 minutes until heated through.

9. Garnish and Serve:

- Garnish with chopped fresh parsley if desired. Serve the Creamy Garlic Parmesan Chicken hot over rice, pasta, or with your favorite side.

Nutritional Information (per serving):

- Calories: 450 kcal
- Protein: 40g
- Fat: 28g
- Carbohydrates: 5g
- Fiber: 1g

Note: Nutritional information is approximate and may vary based on specific ingredients used.

Mushroom and Spinach Stuffed Pork Chops

Prep Time: 20 minutes
Cook Time: 25 minutes
Total Time: 45 minutes
Servings: 4

Ingredients:
For Stuffed Pork Chops:

- 4 thick-cut boneless pork chops
- Salt and black pepper to taste
- 1 tablespoon olive oil
- 2 cups baby spinach, chopped
- 1 cup mushrooms, finely chopped
- 3 cloves garlic, minced
- 1/2 cup shredded mozzarella cheese
- 1/4 cup grated Parmesan cheese

For Seasoning:
- 1 teaspoon dried thyme
- 1 teaspoon dried rosemary
- 1 teaspoon paprika

For Pan Sauce (Optional):
- 1 cup chicken broth
- 2 tablespoons butter
- 2 tablespoons all-purpose flour
- Salt and black pepper to taste

Instructions:

Prepare Stuffed Pork Chops:

1. Preheat Oven:
   - Preheat the oven to 375°F (190°C).

2. Create Pocket in Pork Chops:
   - Using a sharp knife, create a pocket in each pork chop by making a horizontal cut through the center, being careful not to cut all the way through.

3. Season and Stuff:
   - Season the pork chops with salt, black pepper, dried thyme, dried rosemary, and paprika. In a skillet, heat olive oil over medium heat. Sauté chopped spinach, mushrooms, and minced garlic until the spinach wilts and the mushrooms release their moisture. Remove from heat and let it cool slightly. Stuff each pork chop with the spinach and mushroom mixture, then sprinkle with mozzarella and Parmesan cheese.

4. Secure with Toothpicks:
   - Secure the stuffed pork chops with toothpicks to keep the filling in place.

5. Sear Pork Chops:
   - In the same skillet, sear the stuffed pork chops for 2-3 minutes on each side until browned.

6. Bake:
   - Transfer the seared pork chops to a baking dish and bake in the preheated oven for 20-25 minutes

or until the internal temperature reaches 145°F (63°C).

 Prepare Pan Sauce (Optional):
1. Deglaze Skillet:
 - In the same skillet used for searing, deglaze with chicken broth, scraping up any browned bits from the bottom.

2. Make Roux:
 - In a small bowl, mix flour and butter to create a roux. Whisk the roux into the chicken broth and bring to a simmer. Cook until the sauce thickens. Season with salt and black pepper to taste.

3. Serve:
 - Serve the stuffed pork chops with the optional pan sauce drizzled over the top.

 Nutritional Information (per serving, without pan sauce):

- Calories: 400 kcal
- Protein: 40g
- Fat: 20g
- Carbohydrates: 8g
- Fiber: 2g
Note: Nutritional information is approximate and may vary based on specific ingredients used.

Shrimp Scampi with Zoodles

Prep Time: 15 minutes
Cook Time: 10 minutes
Total Time: 25 minutes
Servings: 4

Ingredients:

- 1-pound large shrimp, peeled and deveined
- Salt and black pepper to taste
- 2 tablespoons olive oil
- 4 cloves garlic, minced
- 1/2 teaspoon red pepper flakes (optional)
- 1/2 cup chicken broth
- 1/4 cup dry white wine (or chicken broth)
- Juice of 1 lemon
- Zest of 1 lemon
- 4 medium zucchini, spiralized into zoodles
- 2 tablespoons unsalted butter
- 2 tablespoons chopped fresh parsley
- Grated Parmesan cheese for garnish (optional)

Instructions:

1. Prepare Shrimp:
   - Season the shrimp with salt and black pepper.

2. Cook Shrimp:
     - In a large skillet, heat olive oil over medium-high heat. Add the shrimp and cook for 1-2

minutes on each side until they turn pink. Remove the shrimp from the skillet and set aside.

3. Sauté Garlic and Red Pepper Flakes:
   - In the same skillet, add minced garlic and red pepper flakes (if using). Sauté for about 1 minute until the garlic becomes fragrant.

4. Deglaze with Liquid:
   - Pour in chicken broth and white wine (or additional chicken broth), scraping up any browned bits from the bottom of the skillet.

5. Add Lemon Juice and Zest:
   - Stir in lemon juice and lemon zest, allowing the flavors to meld.

6. Cook Zoodles:
   - Add spiralized zucchini (zoodles) to the skillet and toss until they are just tender, about 2-3 minutes.

7. Finish Dish:
   - Return the cooked shrimp to the skillet. Add butter and chopped parsley. Toss everything together until the shrimp are reheated and the zoodles are coated in the sauce.

8. Serve:
   - Divide the Shrimp Scampi with Zoodles among plates. Garnish with grated Parmesan cheese if desired.

Nutritional Information (per serving):

- Calories: 250 kcal
- Protein: 25g
- Fat: 12g
- Carbohydrates: 10g
- Fiber: 3g

Note: Nutritional information is approximate and may vary based on specific ingredients used.

Brussels Sprouts and Bacon Skillet

Prep Time: 10 minutes
Cook Time: 20 minutes
Total Time: 30 minutes
Servings: 4

Ingredients:

- 1 pound Brussels sprouts, trimmed and halved
- 6 slices bacon, chopped
- 1 tablespoon olive oil
- 2 cloves garlic, minced
- Salt and black pepper to taste
- 1/4 cup chicken broth
- 1 tablespoon balsamic vinegar
- 2 tablespoons grated Parmesan cheese (optional)
- Chopped fresh parsley for garnish (optional)

Instructions:

1. Prepare Brussels Sprouts:
    - Trim the ends of the Brussels sprouts and cut them in half.

2. Cook Bacon:
    - In a large skillet, cook chopped bacon over medium heat until crispy. Remove bacon and set aside, leaving the bacon fat in the skillet.

3. Sauté Brussels Sprouts:

- Add olive oil to the skillet with bacon fat. Add Brussels sprouts and minced garlic. Season with salt and black pepper. Sauté for 5-7 minutes until the sprouts start to brown.

4. Deglaze with Broth:
   - Pour in chicken broth to deglaze the skillet, scraping up any browned bits from the bottom.

5. Finish Cooking:
   - Continue cooking the Brussels sprouts for an additional 5-7 minutes until they are tender but still have a slight bite.

6. Add Bacon and Balsamic Vinegar:
   - Add the cooked bacon back to the skillet. Drizzle balsamic vinegar over the Brussels sprouts and bacon. Toss to coat evenly.

7. Garnish and Serve:
   - Garnish with grated Parmesan cheese and chopped fresh parsley if desired. Serve the Brussels Sprouts and Bacon Skillet hot.

Nutritional Information (per serving):

- Calories: 200 kcal
- Protein: 8g
- Fat: 14g
- Carbohydrates: 12g
- Fiber: 4g

Note: Nutritional information is approximate and may vary based on specific ingredients used.

Chicken Alfredo with Spaghetti Squash

Prep Time: 15 minutes
Cook Time: 45 minutes
Total Time: 1 hour
Servings: 4

Ingredients:

For Spaghetti Squash:

- 1 large spaghetti squash
- 1 tablespoon olive oil
- Salt and black pepper to taste

For Chicken Alfredo:

- 2 boneless, skinless chicken breasts, thinly sliced
- 2 tablespoons unsalted butter
- 2 cloves garlic, minced
- 1 cup heavy cream
- 1 cup grated Parmesan cheese
- Salt and black pepper to taste
- 1/2 teaspoon nutmeg (optional)
- Chopped fresh parsley for garnish (optional)

Instructions:

For Spaghetti Squash:

1. Preheat Oven:
   - Preheat the oven to 375°F (190°C).

2. Prepare Squash:
   - Cut the spaghetti squash in half lengthwise. Scoop out the seeds. Brush the cut sides with olive oil and season with salt and black pepper.

3. Roast Squash:
   - Place the squash halves, cut side down, on a baking sheet. Roast in the preheated oven for 40-45 minutes, or until the flesh is tender and easily scraped with a fork.

4. Scrape and Serve:
   - Scrape the spaghetti squash with a fork to create "noodles." Set aside.

For Chicken Alfredo:

1. Cook Chicken:
   - In a large skillet, heat butter over medium-high heat. Add sliced chicken and cook until browned and cooked through. Remove the chicken from the skillet and set aside.

2. Prepare Alfredo Sauce:
   - In the same skillet, add minced garlic and sauté for 1-2 minutes until fragrant. Pour in heavy cream, grated Parmesan cheese, salt, black pepper, and nutmeg if using. Stir continuously until the cheese is melted and the sauce is smooth.

3. Combine with Spaghetti Squash:

- Add the cooked chicken back to the skillet, tossing to coat in the Alfredo sauce. Add the roasted spaghetti squash noodles and gently combine until everything is well coated.

4. Garnish and Serve:
   - Garnish with chopped fresh parsley if desired. Serve the Chicken Alfredo with Spaghetti Squash hot.

Nutritional Information (per serving):

- Calories: 450 kcal
- Protein: 30g
- Fat: 32g
- Carbohydrates: 15g
- Fiber: 4g

Note: Nutritional information is approximate and may vary based on specific ingredients used.

Turkey and Vegetable Stir-Fry

Prep Time: 15 minutes
Cook Time: 15 minutes
Total Time: 30 minutes
Servings: 4

Ingredients:

For Turkey Marinade:
- 1 pound turkey breast or ground turkey
- 2 tablespoons soy sauce
- 1 tablespoon oyster sauce
- 1 tablespoon cornstarch
- 1 teaspoon sesame oil
- 1 teaspoon ginger, minced
- 1 teaspoon garlic, minced

For Stir-Fry:
- 2 tablespoons vegetable oil
- 1 bell pepper, thinly sliced
- 1 carrot, julienned
- 1 cup broccoli florets
- 1 cup snow peas, ends trimmed
- 3 green onions, sliced
- 1 tablespoon soy sauce
- 1 tablespoon oyster sauce
- 1 teaspoon hoisin sauce
- 1 teaspoon sesame oil
- 1 teaspoon cornstarch mixed with 2 tablespoons water (for thickening)
- Sesame seeds for garnish (optional)

- Cooked brown rice for serving

Instructions:
For Turkey Marinade:

1. Prepare Turkey:
   - If using turkey breast, slice it thinly. If using ground turkey, break it into small pieces.

2. Marinate Turkey:
   - In a bowl, combine soy sauce, oyster sauce, cornstarch, sesame oil, minced ginger, and minced garlic. Add the sliced turkey and marinate for at least 15 minutes.

For Stir-Fry:

1. Heat Oil:
   - In a wok or large skillet, heat vegetable oil over medium-high heat.

2. Cook Turkey:
   - Add the marinated turkey to the hot wok and stir-fry until cooked through and browned. Remove the turkey from the wok and set aside.

3. Stir-Fry Vegetables:
   - In the same wok, add a bit more oil if needed. Stir-fry bell pepper, carrot, broccoli, and snow peas until they are crisp-tender.

4. Combine Turkey and Vegetables:

- Return the cooked turkey to the wok with the vegetables.

5. Prepare Sauce:
   - In a small bowl, mix soy sauce, oyster sauce, hoisin sauce, sesame oil, and the cornstarch-water mixture. Pour the sauce over the turkey and vegetables.

6. Toss and Thicken:
   - Toss everything together until the sauce thickens and coats the turkey and vegetables evenly.

7. Garnish and Serve:
   - Garnish with sliced green onions and sesame seeds if desired. Serve the Turkey and Vegetable Stir-Fry over cooked brown rice.

Nutritional Information (per serving, excluding rice):

- Calories: 250 kcal
- Protein: 25g
- Fat: 12g
- Carbohydrates: 15g
- Fiber: 4g

Note: Nutritional information is approximate and may vary based on specific ingredients used.

Lemon Herb Grilled Swordfish

Prep Time: 15 minutes
Marinating Time: 30 minutes
Cook Time: 8-10 minutes
Total Time: 55 minutes
Servings: 4

Ingredients:

For Swordfish Marinade:

- 4 swordfish steaks (about 6 ounces each)
- 2 tablespoons olive oil
- Zest and juice of 1 lemon
- 2 cloves garlic, minced
- 1 tablespoon fresh parsley, chopped
- 1 teaspoon fresh thyme, chopped
- 1 teaspoon fresh rosemary, chopped
- Salt and black pepper to taste

For Grilling:

- Additional olive oil for brushing grill grates
- Lemon wedges for serving

Instructions:

For Swordfish Marinade:

1. Prepare Swordfish:
   - Pat the swordfish steaks dry with paper towels.

2. Mix Marinade:
  - In a bowl, whisk together olive oil, lemon zest, lemon juice, minced garlic, chopped parsley, chopped thyme, chopped rosemary, salt, and black pepper.

3. Marinate Swordfish:
  - Place the swordfish steaks in a shallow dish and pour the marinade over them. Ensure the steaks are well-coated. Cover the dish and let it marinate in the refrigerator for at least 30 minutes.

 For Grilling:

1. Preheat Grill:
  - Preheat the grill to medium-high heat. Brush the grill grates with olive oil to prevent sticking.

2. Grill Swordfish:
  - Remove the swordfish from the marinade and let any excess drip off. Place the steaks on the preheated grill and cook for 4-5 minutes per side, or until the fish easily flakes with a fork. Cooking time may vary depending on the thickness of the steaks.

3. Baste with Marinade (Optional):
  - Optionally, baste the swordfish with some of the reserved marinade during grilling.

4. Serve:
  - Transfer the grilled swordfish steaks to a serving platter. Serve with lemon wedges on the side.

Nutritional Information (per serving):

- Calories: 300 kcal
- Protein: 35g
- Fat: 15g
- Carbohydrates: 2g
- Fiber: 1g

Note: Nutritional information is approximate and may vary based on specific ingredients used.

Cabbage Roll Casserole

Prep Time: 30 minutes
Cook Time: 1 hour
Total Time: 1 hour 30 minutes
Servings: 6

Ingredients:

For Cabbage and Filling:

- 1 large head of green cabbage
- 1 pound ground beef
- 1 cup cooked rice
- 1 onion, finely chopped
- 2 cloves garlic, minced
- 1 can (14 ounces) crushed tomatoes
- 1 can (8 ounces) tomato sauce
- 1/4 cup tomato paste
- 1/4 cup beef broth
- 1 teaspoon dried oregano
- 1 teaspoon dried basil
- 1 teaspoon paprika
- Salt and black pepper to taste

For Topping:

- 1 cup shredded mozzarella cheese
- Fresh parsley, chopped, for garnish (optional)

Instructions:

For Cabbage and Filling:

1. Precook Cabbage:
   - Preheat the oven to 375°F (190°C). Bring a large pot of water to a boil. Carefully remove the core from the cabbage and place the whole head in the boiling water. Cook for 8-10 minutes until the outer leaves are softened. Remove and let it cool. Peel off the softened leaves and set aside.

2. Prepare Filling:
   - In a skillet, brown the ground beef over medium heat. Add chopped onions and garlic, cooking until the onions are translucent. Drain any excess fat.

3. Combine Ingredients:
   - In a large bowl, mix the cooked rice, browned beef mixture, crushed tomatoes, tomato sauce, tomato paste, beef broth, oregano, basil, paprika, salt, and black pepper.

For Assembly and Baking:

1. Layer Casserole:
   - In a baking dish, spread a thin layer of the beef and rice mixture. Place a layer of cabbage leaves over the mixture. Repeat the process until all the filling and cabbage leaves are used, finishing with a layer of the beef mixture on top.

2. Cover and Bake:
   - Cover the baking dish with aluminum foil and bake in the preheated oven for 45 minutes.

3. Add Cheese Topping:
   - Remove the foil, sprinkle shredded mozzarella cheese over the top, and bake for an additional 15 minutes or until the cheese is melted and bubbly.

4. Garnish and Serve:
   - Remove from the oven and let it rest for a few minutes. Garnish with chopped fresh parsley if desired. Serve the Cabbage Roll Casserole hot.

Nutritional Information (per serving):

- Calories: 350 kcal
- Protein: 20g
- Fat: 15g
- Carbohydrates: 30g
- Fiber: 5g

Note: Nutritional information is approximate and may vary based on specific ingredients used.

Baked Garlic Butter Salmon

Prep Time: 10 minutes
Marinating Time: 30 minutes (optional)
Cook Time: 15 minutes
Total Time: 55 minutes (including marinating time)
Servings: 4

Ingredients:

- 4 salmon fillets (about 6 ounces each)
- 4 tablespoons unsalted butter, melted
- 4 cloves garlic, minced
- 1 tablespoon fresh parsley, chopped
- 1 tablespoon fresh lemon juice
- 1 teaspoon Dijon mustard
- Salt and black pepper to taste
- Lemon slices for garnish
- Chopped fresh parsley for garnish

Instructions:

1. Preheat Oven:
   - Preheat the oven to 375°F (190°C). Line a baking sheet with parchment paper.

2. Prepare Salmon:
   - Pat the salmon fillets dry with paper towels. Place them on the prepared baking sheet.

3. Marinate (Optional):

- In a bowl, mix melted butter, minced garlic, chopped parsley, lemon juice, Dijon mustard, salt, and black pepper. If time allows, you can marinate the salmon in this mixture for 30 minutes in the refrigerator.

4. Brush with Garlic Butter:
   - If not marinating, brush the salmon fillets with the garlic butter mixture, ensuring they are well-coated.

5. Bake:
   - Bake in the preheated oven for 12-15 minutes, or until the salmon flakes easily with a fork. Cooking time may vary based on the thickness of the fillets.

6. Broil (Optional):
   - If desired, broil for an additional 2-3 minutes to give the top a nice golden finish.

7. Garnish and Serve:
   - Garnish the baked salmon with lemon slices and chopped fresh parsley. Serve hot.

Nutritional Information (per serving):

- Calories: 350 kcal
- Protein: 30g
- Fat: 24g
- Carbohydrates: 2g
- Fiber: 0g

Note: Nutritional information is approximate and
may vary based on specific ingredients used.

Sausage and Cauliflower Rice Skillet

Prep Time: 15 minutes
Cook Time: 20 minutes
Total Time: 35 minutes
Servings: 4

Ingredients:

- 1 pound ground sausage (mild or hot, based on preference)
- 1 medium-sized cauliflower, riced
- 1 bell pepper, diced
- 1 onion, finely chopped
- 2 cloves garlic, minced
- 1 can (14 ounces) diced tomatoes, drained
- 1 teaspoon Italian seasoning
- 1/2 teaspoon paprika
- Salt and black pepper to taste
- 1 cup shredded mozzarella cheese
- Fresh parsley, chopped, for garnish (optional)

Instructions:

1. Prepare Cauliflower Rice:
   - Cut the cauliflower into florets and use a food processor to rice it. Alternatively, you can use a box grater.

2. Cook Sausage:

- In a large skillet, cook the ground sausage over medium-high heat until browned. Break it apart with a spoon as it cooks.

3. Add Vegetables:
   - Add diced bell pepper, chopped onion, and minced garlic to the skillet. Sauté until the vegetables are tender.

4. Stir in Cauliflower Rice:
   - Stir in the riced cauliflower and cook for 5-7 minutes, or until the cauliflower is cooked through and slightly golden.

5. Season:
   - Season the mixture with Italian seasoning, paprika, salt, and black pepper. Mix well to combine.

6. Add Tomatoes:
   - Add the drained diced tomatoes to the skillet and stir to incorporate.

7. Top with Cheese:
   - Sprinkle shredded mozzarella cheese over the top of the skillet. Cover the skillet and let it melt for a few minutes.

8. Garnish and Serve:
   - Once the cheese is melted and bubbly, garnish with chopped fresh parsley if desired. Serve the Sausage and Cauliflower Rice Skillet hot.

Nutritional Information (per serving):

- Calories: 380 kcal
- Protein: 18g
- Fat: 30g
- Carbohydrates: 10g
- Fiber: 4g

Note: Nutritional information is approximate and may vary based on specific ingredients used.

Chicken and Broccoli Alfredo Bake

Prep Time: 20 minutes
Cook Time: 25 minutes
Total Time: 45 minutes
Servings: 6

Ingredients:

- 1-pound boneless, skinless chicken breasts, cooked and shredded
- 1 pound broccoli florets, steamed
- 1 pound penne pasta, cooked according to package instructions
- 2 cups shredded mozzarella cheese
- 1 cup grated Parmesan cheese
- 1/2 cup unsalted butter
- 1 cup heavy cream
- 4 cloves garlic, minced
- 1 teaspoon dried oregano
- 1 teaspoon dried basil
- Salt and black pepper to taste
- Fresh parsley, chopped, for garnish (optional)

Instructions:

1. Preheat Oven:
   - Preheat the oven to 375°F (190°C). Grease a 9x13-inch baking dish.

2. Prepare Chicken and Broccoli:

- Cook and shred the chicken breasts. Steam the broccoli florets until tender. Cook the penne pasta according to package instructions.

3. Make Alfredo Sauce:
   - In a saucepan, melt the butter over medium heat. Add minced garlic and sauté until fragrant. Pour in the heavy cream, dried oregano, dried basil, salt, and black pepper. Stir and simmer until the sauce thickens.

4. Assemble Bake:
   - In the prepared baking dish, combine the cooked and shredded chicken, steamed broccoli, and cooked penne pasta. Pour the Alfredo sauce over the mixture and toss until everything is well coated.

5. Add Cheese:
   - Sprinkle shredded mozzarella and grated Parmesan cheese over the top of the pasta mixture.

6. Bake:
   - Bake in the preheated oven for 20-25 minutes, or until the cheese is melted and bubbly, and the edges are golden brown.

7. Garnish and Serve:
   - Remove from the oven, garnish with chopped fresh parsley if desired, and serve the Chicken and Broccoli Alfredo Bake hot.

Nutritional Information (per serving):

- Calories: 580 kcal
- Protein: 30g
- Fat: 35g
- Carbohydrates: 42g
- Fiber: 4g

Note: Nutritional information is approximate and may vary based on specific ingredients used.

Pesto Zoodle Bowl with Grilled Chicken

Prep Time: 20 minutes
Marinating Time: 30 minutes
Cook Time: 10 minutes
Total Time: 1 hour
Servings: 4

Ingredients:

For Grilled Chicken:

- 1.5 pounds boneless, skinless chicken breasts
- 2 tablespoons olive oil
- 2 cloves garlic, minced
- 1 tablespoon lemon juice
- 1 teaspoon dried basil
- 1 teaspoon dried oregano
- Salt and black pepper to taste

For Pesto Zoodles:

- 4 medium zucchini, spiralized into zoodles
- 1 cup cherry tomatoes, halved
- 1/2 cup black olives, sliced
- 1/2 cup feta cheese, crumbled
- Fresh basil leaves for garnish (optional)

For Pesto Sauce:

- 2 cups fresh basil leaves
- 1/2 cup pine nuts

- 1/2 cup grated Parmesan cheese
- 2 cloves garlic, minced
- 1/2 cup extra-virgin olive oil
- Salt and black pepper to taste
- Juice of 1 lemon

Instructions:

For Grilled Chicken:

1. Marinate Chicken:
   - In a bowl, mix olive oil, minced garlic, lemon juice, dried basil, dried oregano, salt, and black pepper. Coat the chicken breasts with the marinade and let them marinate in the refrigerator for at least 30 minutes.

2. Grill Chicken:
   - Preheat the grill. Grill the marinated chicken breasts for 4-5 minutes per side, or until fully cooked and grill marks appear. Let them rest for a few minutes before slicing.

For Pesto Zoodles:

1. Prepare Pesto Sauce:
   - In a food processor, combine fresh basil, pine nuts, grated Parmesan cheese, minced garlic, olive oil, salt, black pepper, and lemon juice. Blend until smooth.

2. Assemble Zoodle Bowl:

- In a large bowl, toss the spiralized zucchini with the pesto sauce until well coated. Add cherry tomatoes, black olives, and crumbled feta cheese. Mix gently.

3. Serve:
- Divide the pesto zoodles among serving plates. Top with grilled chicken slices. Garnish with fresh basil leaves if desired. Serve the Pesto Zoodle Bowl with Grilled Chicken immediately.

Nutritional Information (per serving):

- Calories: 450 kcal
- Protein: 35g
- Fat: 30g
- Carbohydrates: 12g
- Fiber: 4g

Note: Nutritional information is approximate and may vary based on specific ingredients used.

Beef and Vegetable Kebabs

Prep Time: 20 minutes
Marinating Time: 2 hours (or overnight)
Cook Time: 15 minutes
Total Time: 2 hours 35 minutes
Servings: 4

Ingredients:

For Marinade:

- 1.5 pounds sirloin or top sirloin steak, cut into 1-inch cubes
- 1/4 cup soy sauce
- 2 tablespoons olive oil
- 2 tablespoons balsamic vinegar
- 2 cloves garlic, minced
- 1 teaspoon dried rosemary
- 1 teaspoon dried thyme
- 1 teaspoon smoked paprika
- Salt and black pepper to taste

For Kebabs:

- 1 red bell pepper, cut into chunks
- 1 yellow bell pepper, cut into chunks
- 1 red onion, cut into chunks
- 1 zucchini, sliced into rounds
- Cherry tomatoes
- Wooden or metal skewers

Instructions:

For Marinade:

1. Prepare Marinade:
   - In a bowl, whisk together soy sauce, olive oil, balsamic vinegar, minced garlic, dried rosemary, dried thyme, smoked paprika, salt, and black pepper.

2. Marinate Beef:
   - Place the cubed steak in a resealable plastic bag or shallow dish. Pour the marinade over the beef, ensuring it is well-coated. Seal the bag or cover the dish and let it marinate in the refrigerator for at least 2 hours, or preferably overnight.

For Kebabs:

1. Preheat Grill:
   - Preheat the grill to medium-high heat.

2. Assemble Kebabs:
   - Remove the marinated beef from the refrigerator. Thread the marinated beef, bell pepper chunks, red onion chunks, zucchini slices, and cherry tomatoes onto the skewers, alternating between the ingredients.

3. Grill Kebabs:
   - Place the assembled kebabs on the preheated grill. Grill for about 10-15 minutes, turning

occasionally, until the beef reaches your desired level of doneness and the vegetables are tender.

4. Serve:
   - Remove the kebabs from the grill and let them rest for a few minutes. Serve the Beef and Vegetable Kebabs hot.

Nutritional Information (per serving):

- Calories: 350 kcal
- Protein: 30g
- Fat: 18g
- Carbohydrates: 15g
- Fiber: 4g

Note: Nutritional information is approximate and may vary based on specific ingredients used.

Cajun Shrimp and Sausage Sheet Pan Dinner

Prep Time: 15 minutes
Cook Time: 20 minutes
Total Time: 35 minutes
Servings: 4

Ingredients:

- 1-pound large shrimp, peeled and deveined
- 12 ounces andouille sausage, sliced
- 1 pound baby potatoes, halved
- 1 red bell pepper, sliced
- 1 yellow bell pepper, sliced
- 1 red onion, sliced
- 3 tablespoons olive oil
- 2 tablespoons Cajun seasoning
- 1 teaspoon smoked paprika
- 1 teaspoon dried thyme
- 1 teaspoon garlic powder
- Salt and black pepper to taste
- Fresh parsley, chopped, for garnish
- Lemon wedges for serving

Instructions:

1. Preheat Oven:
   - Preheat the oven to 425°F (220°C). Line a large baking sheet with parchment paper.

2. Prepare Ingredients:

   - In a large bowl, combine shrimp, sliced andouille sausage, halved baby potatoes, sliced red and yellow bell peppers, and sliced red onion.

3. Make Cajun Seasoning:
   - In a small bowl, mix together olive oil, Cajun seasoning, smoked paprika, dried thyme, garlic powder, salt, and black pepper.

4. Coat Ingredients:
   - Pour the Cajun seasoning mixture over the shrimp, sausage, and vegetables. Toss everything together until well coated.

5. Arrange on Baking Sheet:
   - Spread the seasoned shrimp, sausage, and vegetables in an even layer on the prepared baking sheet.

6. Roast in Oven:
   - Roast in the preheated oven for 18-20 minutes, or until the shrimp are opaque, the sausage is browned, and the potatoes are tender.

7. Garnish and Serve:
   - Remove from the oven, garnish with chopped fresh parsley, and serve the Cajun Shrimp and Sausage Sheet Pan Dinner hot. Serve with lemon wedges for a burst of citrus flavor.

Nutritional Information (per serving):

- Calories: 480 kcal

- Protein: 30g
- Fat: 25g
- Carbohydrates: 35g
- Fiber: 5g

Note: Nutritional information is approximate and may vary based on specific ingredients used.

Eggplant Lasagna Roll-Ups

Prep Time: 30 minutes
Cook Time: 40 minutes
Total Time: 1 hour 10 minutes
Servings: 4

Ingredients:

For Eggplant "Noodles":
- 2 large eggplants, thinly sliced lengthwise
- 2 tablespoons olive oil
- Salt and black pepper to taste

For Filling:
- 1 cup ricotta cheese
- 1 cup shredded mozzarella cheese
- 1/2 cup grated Parmesan cheese
- 1 large egg
- 2 tablespoons fresh basil, chopped
- 2 tablespoons fresh parsley, chopped
- 1 teaspoon garlic powder
- Salt and black pepper to taste

For Assembly:

- 2 cups marinara sauce
- 1 cup shredded mozzarella cheese
- Fresh basil leaves for garnish (optional)

Instructions:

For Eggplant "Noodles":

1. Preheat Oven:
   - Preheat the oven to 375°F (190°C).

2. Prepare Eggplant:
   - Slice the eggplants lengthwise into thin strips. Place the slices on a baking sheet, brush with olive oil, and season with salt and black pepper.

3. Roast Eggplant:
   - Roast the eggplant slices in the preheated oven for 15-20 minutes or until softened. Remove from the oven and set aside.

For Filling:

1. Make Filling:
   - In a bowl, combine ricotta cheese, shredded mozzarella cheese, grated Parmesan cheese, egg, chopped fresh basil, chopped fresh parsley, garlic powder, salt, and black pepper. Mix until well combined.

For Assembly:

1. Assemble Roll-Ups:
   - Take a roasted eggplant slice and spoon some of the cheese filling onto one end. Roll it up and place it seam-side down in a baking dish. Repeat with the remaining eggplant slices and filling.

2. Top with Marinara Sauce:

- Pour marinara sauce over the eggplant roll-ups, ensuring they are well-covered.

3. Add Cheese:
   - Sprinkle shredded mozzarella cheese over the top.

4. Bake:
   - Bake in the preheated oven for 20-25 minutes or until the cheese is melted and bubbly.

5. Garnish and Serve:
   - Remove from the oven, garnish with fresh basil leaves if desired, and serve the Eggplant Lasagna Roll-Ups hot.

Nutritional Information (per serving):

- Calories: 380 kcal
- Protein: 20g
- Fat: 28g
- Carbohydrates: 20g
- Fiber: 8g

Note: Nutritional information is approximate and may vary based on specific ingredients used.

Greek Lamb Chops with Tzatziki

Prep Time: 15 minutes
Marinating Time: 2 hours (or overnight)
Cook Time: 15 minutes

Total Time: 2 hours 30 minutes
Servings: 4

Ingredients:

For Lamb Chops:

- 8 lamb chops
- 2 tablespoons olive oil
- 3 cloves garlic, minced
- 1 tablespoon fresh rosemary, chopped
- 1 tablespoon fresh oregano, chopped
- 1 teaspoon dried thyme
- Juice of 1 lemon
- Salt and black pepper to taste

For Tzatziki:

- 1 cup Greek yogurt
- 1 cucumber, finely diced
- 2 cloves garlic, minced
- 1 tablespoon fresh dill, chopped
- 1 tablespoon fresh mint, chopped
- 1 tablespoon olive oil
- Juice of 1/2 lemon
- Salt and black pepper to taste

Instructions:

For Lamb Chops:

1. Marinate Lamb Chops:

- In a bowl, mix olive oil, minced garlic, chopped rosemary, chopped oregano, dried thyme, lemon juice, salt, and black pepper. Coat the lamb chops with the marinade and let them marinate in the refrigerator for at least 2 hours, or preferably overnight.

2. Preheat Grill or Pan:
   - Preheat the grill or a grill pan to medium-high heat.

3. Grill Lamb Chops:
   - Grill the marinated lamb chops for 5-7 minutes per side, or until they reach your desired level of doneness. Cooking time may vary based on thickness.

For Tzatziki:

1. Prepare Tzatziki:
   - In a bowl, combine Greek yogurt, finely diced cucumber, minced garlic, chopped fresh dill, chopped fresh mint, olive oil, lemon juice, salt, and black pepper. Mix well.

2. Serve:
   - Serve the grilled Greek Lamb Chops with a side of Tzatziki sauce.

Nutritional Information (per serving):

- Calories: 450 kcal
- Protein: 35g

- Fat: 30g
- Carbohydrates: 10g
- Fiber: 2g

Note: Nutritional information is approximate and may vary based on specific ingredients used.

Cauliflower Shepherd's Pie

Prep Time: 20 minutes
Cook Time: 30 minutes
Total Time: 50 minutes
Servings: 6

Ingredients:

For Cauliflower Mash:

- 1 large head cauliflower, cut into florets
- 2 tablespoons butter
- 1/4 cup heavy cream
- Salt and black pepper to taste

For Filling:

- 1 tablespoon olive oil
- 1 onion, diced
- 2 carrots, diced
- 2 cloves garlic, minced
- 1.5 pounds ground lamb or beef
- 2 tablespoons tomato paste
- 1 cup frozen peas
- 1 cup beef or vegetable broth
- 1 tablespoon Worcestershire sauce
- 1 teaspoon dried thyme
- Salt and black pepper to taste

Instructions:

For Cauliflower Mash:

1. Steam Cauliflower:
   - Steam the cauliflower florets until tender.

2. Make Cauliflower Mash:
   - In a blender or food processor, combine steamed cauliflower, butter, heavy cream, salt, and black pepper. Blend until smooth and creamy. Set aside.

For Filling:

1. Sauté Vegetables:
   - In a large skillet, heat olive oil over medium heat. Sauté diced onion and carrots until softened.

2. Cook Ground Meat:
   - Add minced garlic and ground lamb or beef to the skillet. Cook until the meat is browned.

3. Add Flavorings:
   - Stir in tomato paste, frozen peas, beef or vegetable broth, Worcestershire sauce, dried thyme, salt, and black pepper. Simmer for 10-15 minutes until the mixture thickens.

4. Assemble Shepherd's Pie:
   - Preheat the oven to 400°F (200°C). Transfer the meat mixture to a baking dish. Spread the cauliflower mash evenly over the top.

5. Bake:

  - Bake in the preheated oven for 20 minutes or until the top is golden and the filling is bubbly.

6. Serve:
  - Remove from the oven and let it cool for a few minutes before serving the Cauliflower Shepherd's Pie.

 Nutritional Information (per serving):

- Calories: 320 kcal
- Protein: 20g
- Fat: 20g
- Carbohydrates: 15g
- Fiber: 5g

Note: Nutritional information is approximate and may vary based on specific ingredients used.

Spaghetti Squash Carbonara

Prep Time: 20 minutes
Cook Time: 40 minutes
Total Time: 1 hour
Servings: 4

Ingredients:

- 1 large spaghetti squash
- 2 tablespoons olive oil
- 4 ounces pancetta or bacon, diced
- 3 cloves garlic, minced
- 1/2 cup grated Pecorino Romano cheese
- 1/2 cup grated Parmesan cheese
- 3 large eggs, beaten
- Salt and black pepper to taste
- Fresh parsley, chopped, for garnish

Instructions:

1. Preheat Oven:
   - Preheat the oven to 375°F (190°C).

2. Prepare Spaghetti Squash:
   - Cut the spaghetti squash in half lengthwise and scoop out the seeds. Drizzle the cut sides with olive oil, season with salt and black pepper, and place them cut side down on a baking sheet.

3. Roast Spaghetti Squash:

- Roast the spaghetti squash in the preheated oven for 35-40 minutes or until the flesh is fork-tender. Allow it to cool slightly.

4. Prepare Carbonara Sauce:
   - In a skillet, cook the diced pancetta or bacon over medium heat until crispy. Add minced garlic and sauté for an additional 1-2 minutes.

5. Scrape Squash Strands:
   - Use a fork to scrape the strands from the roasted spaghetti squash and transfer them to a large bowl.

6. Assemble Carbonara:
   - In a separate bowl, mix together the beaten eggs, grated Pecorino Romano cheese, and grated Parmesan cheese.

7. Combine Ingredients:
   - Quickly toss the hot spaghetti squash strands with the egg and cheese mixture. The heat from the squash will cook the eggs and create a creamy sauce. Add the cooked pancetta or bacon and garlic, tossing to combine. Season with salt and black pepper to taste.

8. Serve:
   - Garnish with chopped fresh parsley and serve the Spaghetti Squash Carbonara immediately.

Nutritional Information (per serving):

- Calories: 350 kcal

- Protein: 15g
- Fat: 25g
- Carbohydrates: 20g
- Fiber: 5g

Note: Nutritional information is approximate and may vary based on specific ingredients used.

Lemon Dill Baked Cod

Prep Time: 10 minutes
Marinating Time: 30 minutes
Cook Time: 15 minutes
Total Time: 55 minutes
Servings: 4

Ingredients:

- 4 cod fillets
- 2 tablespoons olive oil
- 2 tablespoons fresh lemon juice
- 1 teaspoon lemon zest
- 2 cloves garlic, minced
- 2 tablespoons fresh dill, chopped
- Salt and black pepper to taste
- Lemon slices for garnish

Instructions:

1. Marinate Cod:
   - In a bowl, whisk together olive oil, fresh lemon juice, lemon zest, minced garlic, chopped fresh dill, salt, and black pepper. Place the cod fillets in a shallow dish and pour the marinade over them. Let it marinate for at least 30 minutes in the refrigerator.

2. Preheat Oven:
   - Preheat the oven to 400°F (200°C).

3. Bake Cod:
   - Place the marinated cod fillets on a baking sheet lined with parchment paper. Bake in the preheated oven for 12-15 minutes or until the cod flakes easily with a fork.

4. Broil for Crispy Top (Optional):
   - If desired, broil the cod for an additional 2-3 minutes to get a slightly crispy top.

5. Garnish and Serve:
   - Garnish with additional fresh dill and lemon slices. Serve the Lemon Dill Baked Cod hot.

Nutritional Information (per serving):

- Calories: 200 kcal
- Protein: 25g
- Fat: 9g
- Carbohydrates: 2g
- Fiber: 0g

Note: Nutritional information is approximate and may vary based on specific ingredients used.

Broccoli Cheddar Stuffed Chicken Breast

Prep Time: 20 minutes
Cook Time: 25 minutes
Total Time: 45 minutes
Servings: 4

Ingredients:

- 4 boneless, skinless chicken breasts
- 1 cup broccoli florets, steamed and chopped
- 1 cup shredded cheddar cheese
- 2 tablespoons cream cheese, softened
- 2 cloves garlic, minced
- 1 teaspoon dried thyme
- 1 teaspoon paprika
- Salt and black pepper to taste
- 2 tablespoons olive oil
- Chopped fresh parsley for garnish

Instructions:

1. Preheat Oven:
   - Preheat the oven to 400°F (200°C).

2. Prepare Chicken Breasts:
   - Place each chicken breast between sheets of plastic wrap and use a meat mallet to pound them to an even thickness.

3. Make Filling:

- In a bowl, mix together chopped broccoli, shredded cheddar cheese, softened cream cheese, minced garlic, dried thyme, paprika, salt, and black pepper.

4. Stuff Chicken Breasts:
   - Divide the broccoli and cheddar filling evenly among the chicken breasts. Fold the chicken over the filling and secure with toothpicks if needed.

5. Season Chicken:
   - Season the stuffed chicken breasts with additional salt, pepper, and paprika.

6. Sear Chicken:
   - In an oven-safe skillet, heat olive oil over medium-high heat. Sear the stuffed chicken breasts for 2-3 minutes on each side until golden brown.

7. Bake:
   - Transfer the skillet to the preheated oven and bake for 20-25 minutes or until the chicken is cooked through.

8. Garnish and Serve:
   - Garnish with chopped fresh parsley and serve the Broccoli Cheddar Stuffed Chicken Breast hot.

Nutritional Information (per serving):

- Calories: 350 kcal
- Protein: 35g

- Fat: 20g
- Carbohydrates: 5g
- Fiber: 2g

Note: Nutritional information is approximate and may vary based on specific ingredients used.

Tomato Basil Mozzarella Chicken

Prep Time: 15 minutes
Cook Time: 25 minutes
Total Time: 40 minutes
Servings: 4

Ingredients:

- 4 boneless, skinless chicken breasts
- Salt and black pepper to taste
- 2 tablespoons olive oil
- 4 cloves garlic, minced
- 1 cup cherry tomatoes, halved
- 1/2 cup fresh basil leaves, chopped
- 8 ounces fresh mozzarella cheese, sliced
- Balsamic glaze for drizzling (optional)
- Chopped fresh basil for garnish

Instructions:

1. Preheat Oven:
   - Preheat the oven to 400°F (200°C).

2. Season Chicken:
   - Season chicken breasts with salt and black pepper.

3. Sear Chicken:
   - In an oven-safe skillet, heat olive oil over medium-high heat. Sear the chicken breasts for 2-3 minutes on each side until golden brown.

4. Add Garlic and Tomatoes:
   - Add minced garlic to the skillet and sauté for 1 minute. Add halved cherry tomatoes and cook for an additional 2 minutes.

5. Top with Mozzarella:
   - Place slices of fresh mozzarella on top of each chicken breast.

6. Bake:
   - Transfer the skillet to the preheated oven and bake for 15-20 minutes or until the chicken is cooked through and the cheese is melted and bubbly.

7. Garnish and Serve:
   - Remove from the oven, sprinkle chopped fresh basil over the top, and drizzle with balsamic glaze if desired. Serve the Tomato Basil Mozzarella Chicken hot.

 Nutritional Information (per serving):

- Calories: 350 kcal
- Protein: 40g
- Fat: 18g
- Carbohydrates: 4g
- Fiber: 1g

Note: Nutritional information is approximate and may vary based on specific ingredients used.

Asparagus and Feta Stuffed Turkey Burgers

Prep Time: 15 minutes
Cook Time: 15 minutes
Total Time: 30 minutes
Servings: 4

Ingredients:

For Turkey Patties:

- 1 pound ground turkey
- 1/2 cup breadcrumbs
- 1 egg
- 2 cloves garlic, minced
- 1 teaspoon dried oregano
- Salt and black pepper to taste

For Filling:

- 1 bunch asparagus, blanched and chopped
- 1/2 cup crumbled feta cheese

Additional Ingredients:

- Olive oil for cooking
- Whole wheat burger buns
- Lettuce, tomato, and red onion for garnish

Instructions:

For Turkey Patties:

1. Prepare Turkey Mixture:
   - In a bowl, combine ground turkey, breadcrumbs, egg, minced garlic, dried oregano, salt, and black pepper. Mix until well combined.

2. Form Patties:
   - Divide the turkey mixture into 8 equal portions. Take 4 portions and shape them into thin patties.

For Filling:

1. Assemble Filling:
   - In a small bowl, mix blanched and chopped asparagus with crumbled feta cheese.

2. Add Filling:
   - Spoon the asparagus and feta mixture onto the center of 4 turkey patties.

3. Top with Patties:
   - Place the remaining 4 patties on top and seal the edges, creating stuffed turkey patties.

Cooking:

1. Cook Stuffed Patties:
   - In a skillet, heat olive oil over medium heat. Cook the stuffed turkey patties for about 5-7 minutes per side or until fully cooked.

2. Serve:

- Serve the Asparagus and Feta Stuffed Turkey Burgers on whole wheat buns with lettuce, tomato, and red onion.

 Nutritional Information (per serving, without buns and toppings):

- Calories: 250 kcal
- Protein: 25g
- Fat: 12g
- Carbohydrates: 10g
- Fiber: 2g

Note: Nutritional information is approximate and may vary based on specific ingredients used.

Snacks

Cheese and Pepperoni Roll-Ups

Prep Time: 10 minutes
Cook Time: 10 minutes
Total Time: 20 minutes
Servings: 4

Ingredients:

- 1 package (8 ounces) crescent roll dough
- 1/2 cup shredded mozzarella cheese
- 1/4 cup grated Parmesan cheese
- 1/2 cup pepperoni slices
- 1 teaspoon Italian seasoning
- 1/2 cup pizza sauce for dipping

Instructions:

1. Preheat Oven:
   - Preheat the oven according to the crescent roll package instructions.

2. Prepare Crescent Roll Dough:
   - Roll out the crescent roll dough and separate it into individual triangles.

3. Assemble Roll-Ups:

- Sprinkle each triangle with shredded mozzarella and grated Parmesan cheese. Place a few pepperoni slices on top.

4. Roll Up:
   - Starting from the wide end, roll up each triangle, enclosing the cheese and pepperoni.

5. Place on Baking Sheet:
   - Arrange the roll-ups on a baking sheet lined with parchment paper.

6. Sprinkle with Seasoning:
   - Sprinkle Italian seasoning over the top of each roll-up.

7. Bake:
   - Bake in the preheated oven for the time specified on the crescent roll package or until the roll-ups are golden brown.

8. Serve with Pizza Sauce:
   - Serve the Cheese and Pepperoni Roll-Ups warm with pizza sauce for dipping.

Nutritional Information (per serving):

- Calories: 220 kcal
- Protein: 8g
- Fat: 14g
- Carbohydrates: 15g
- Fiber: 1g

Note: Nutritional information is approximate and may vary based on specific ingredients used.

Avocado and Bacon Deviled Eggs

Prep Time: 20 minutes
Cook Time: 10 minutes (for boiling eggs)
Total Time: 30 minutes
Servings: 6

Ingredients:

- 6 large eggs
- 1 ripe avocado
- 3 slices bacon, cooked and crumbled
- 2 tablespoons mayonnaise
- 1 tablespoon Dijon mustard
- 1 tablespoon fresh lemon juice
- Salt and black pepper to taste
- Chopped chives or paprika for garnish

Instructions:

1. Hard Boil Eggs:
   - Place the eggs in a saucepan and cover them with water. Bring the water to a boil, then reduce the heat and simmer for 10 minutes. Transfer the eggs to an ice bath to cool before peeling.

2. Cut and Scoop Avocado:
   - Cut the avocado in half, remove the pit, and scoop out the flesh into a bowl.

3. Prepare Bacon:

- Cook the bacon until crispy, then crumble it into small pieces.

4. Make Deviled Egg Filling:
   - Slice the hard-boiled eggs in half and carefully remove the yolks. Place the yolks in the bowl with the avocado. Add mayonnaise, Dijon mustard, fresh lemon juice, salt, and black pepper. Mash and mix until smooth.

5. Assemble Deviled Eggs:
   - Spoon or pipe the avocado and yolk mixture back into the egg whites.

6. Top with Bacon:
   - Sprinkle crumbled bacon over the filled eggs.

7. Garnish and Serve:
   - Garnish with chopped chives or a sprinkle of paprika. Serve the Avocado and Bacon Deviled Eggs chilled.

Nutritional Information (per serving, based on 2 halves):

- Calories: 180 kcal
- Protein: 9g
- Fat: 15g
- Carbohydrates: 4g
- Fiber: 2g

Note: Nutritional information is approximate and may vary based on specific ingredients used.

Cucumber and Cream Cheese Bites

Prep Time: 15 minutes
Total Time: 15 minutes
Servings: 4

Ingredients:

- 1 large cucumber
- 1/2 cup cream cheese, softened
- 2 tablespoons fresh dill, chopped
- 1 tablespoon chives, finely chopped
- Salt and black pepper to taste
- Smoked salmon or prosciutto for topping (optional)

Instructions:

1. Prepare Cucumber:
   - Wash the cucumber and cut it into thick slices.

2. Hollow Cucumber Slices:
   - Use a small spoon or melon baller to hollow out the center of each cucumber slice, creating a small well.

3. Make Cream Cheese Mixture:
   - In a bowl, mix the softened cream cheese with chopped fresh dill and chives. Season with salt and black pepper to taste.

4. Fill Cucumber Bites:

- Spoon or pipe the cream cheese mixture into the well of each cucumber slice.

5. Optional Toppings:
  - Top each cucumber and cream cheese bite with a small piece of smoked salmon or prosciutto if desired.

6. Garnish and Serve:
  - Garnish with additional fresh dill or chives. Serve the Cucumber and Cream Cheese Bites chilled.

Nutritional Information (per serving):

- Calories: 90 kcal
- Protein: 2g
- Fat: 8g
- Carbohydrates: 3g
- Fiber: 1g

Note: Nutritional information is approximate and may vary based on specific ingredients used.

Spicy Guacamole with Jicama Sticks

Prep Time: 20 minutes
Total Time: 20 minutes
Servings: 4

Ingredients:

- 3 ripe avocados
- 1 medium tomato, diced
- 1/4 cup red onion, finely chopped
- 1/4 cup fresh cilantro, chopped
- 1 jalapeño, seeds removed and finely diced
- 2 cloves garlic, minced
- Juice of 2 limes
- Salt and black pepper to taste
- Jicama sticks for dipping

Instructions:

1. Prepare Avocados:
   - Cut the avocados in half, remove the pits, and scoop the flesh into a bowl.

2. Mash Avocados:
   - Use a fork to mash the avocados to your desired level of smoothness.

3. Add Ingredients:
   - Add diced tomato, chopped red onion, cilantro, diced jalapeño, minced garlic, and lime juice to the mashed avocados.

4. Mix and Season:
   - Mix all the ingredients together until well combined. Season with salt and black pepper to taste.

5. Chill:
   - If time allows, refrigerate the guacamole for about 15 minutes to let the flavors meld.

6. Serve with Jicama Sticks:
   - Peel the jicama and cut it into sticks for dipping. Serve the Spicy Guacamole with Jicama Sticks.

Nutritional Information (per serving):

- Calories: 200 kcal
- Protein: 3g
- Fat: 16g
- Carbohydrates: 15g
- Fiber: 10g

Note: Nutritional information is approximate and may vary based on specific ingredients used.

Parmesan Crisps

Prep Time: 5 minutes
Cook Time: 7 minutes
Total Time: 12 minutes
Servings: 4

Ingredients:

- 1 cup Parmesan cheese, finely grated
- 1 teaspoon garlic powder (optional)
- 1/2 teaspoon black pepper (optional)
- 1 tablespoon fresh herbs (such as thyme or rosemary), chopped (optional)

Instructions:

1. Preheat Oven:
   - Preheat your oven to 400°F (200°C). Line a baking sheet with parchment paper.

2. Grate Parmesan:
   - Finely grate Parmesan cheese. If desired, mix in garlic powder, black pepper, or fresh herbs for added flavor.

3. Create Mounds:
   - Spoon small mounds (about 1 tablespoon each) of grated Parmesan onto the prepared baking sheet, spacing them apart.

4. Flatten Mounds:

- Gently flatten each mound with the back of a spoon to form thin circles.

5. Bake:
   - Bake in the preheated oven for about 5-7 minutes or until the edges are golden brown.

6. Cool:
  - Allow the Parmesan crisps to cool on the baking sheet for a few minutes. They will continue to firm up as they cool.

7. Serve:
   - Once completely cooled and crisp, carefully remove the Parmesan crisps from the parchment paper. Serve and enjoy!

Note:

- Variations:
  - Experiment with different flavor variations by adding garlic powder, black pepper, or fresh herbs to the grated Parmesan before baking.

Nutritional Information (per serving):

- Calories: 80 kcal
- Protein: 7g
- Fat: 5g
- Carbohydrates: 1g
- Fiber: 0g

Note: Nutritional information is approximate and may vary based on specific ingredients used.

Hard-Boiled Eggs with Dill

Prep Time: 10 minutes
Cook Time: 10 minutes (for boiling eggs)
Total Time: 20 minutes
Servings: 4

Ingredients:

- 6 large eggs
- 2 tablespoons fresh dill, chopped
- 1 tablespoon mayonnaise
- 1 teaspoon Dijon mustard
- Salt and black pepper to taste
- Fresh dill sprigs for garnish (optional)

Instructions:

1. Boil Eggs:
   - Place the eggs in a saucepan and cover them with water. Bring the water to a boil, then reduce the heat and simmer for 10 minutes. Transfer the eggs to an ice bath to cool before peeling.

2. Prepare Egg Mixture:
   - Once the eggs are cooled and peeled, cut them in half lengthwise. Remove the yolks and place them in a bowl.

3. Add Ingredients:
   - To the egg yolks, add chopped fresh dill, mayonnaise, Dijon mustard, salt, and black pepper.

4. Mash and Mix:
   - Mash the egg yolks and mix all the ingredients together until well combined.

5. Fill Egg Whites:
   - Spoon or pipe the dill and egg yolk mixture back into the egg white halves.

6. Garnish and Serve:
   - Garnish with fresh dill sprigs if desired. Serve the Hard-Boiled Eggs with Dill chilled.

 Nutritional Information (per serving, based on 2 halves):

- Calories: 120 kcal
- Protein: 8g
- Fat: 9g
- Carbohydrates: 1g
- Fiber: 0g

Note: Nutritional information is approximate and may vary based on specific ingredients used.

Buffalo Cauliflower Bites

Prep Time: 15 minutes
Cook Time: 25 minutes
Total Time: 40 minutes
Servings: 4

Ingredients:

- 1 medium cauliflower head, cut into florets
- 1 cup all-purpose flour
- 1 cup water
- 1 teaspoon garlic powder
- 1/2 teaspoon onion powder
- 1/2 teaspoon smoked paprika
- 1/4 teaspoon salt
- 1/4 teaspoon black pepper
- 1/2 cup buffalo sauce
- 2 tablespoons unsalted butter, melted
- Ranch or blue cheese dressing for dipping
- Fresh parsley for garnish (optional)

Instructions:

1. Preheat Oven:
    - Preheat the oven to 450°F (230°C). Line a baking sheet with parchment paper.

2. Prepare Batter:
    - In a bowl, whisk together flour, water, garlic powder, onion powder, smoked paprika, salt, and black pepper to create a smooth batter.

3. Coat Cauliflower:
   - Dip each cauliflower floret into the batter, ensuring it's well coated, and place it on the prepared baking sheet.

4. Bake:
   - Bake in the preheated oven for 20-25 minutes or until the cauliflower is golden brown and crispy.

5. Prepare Buffalo Sauce:
   - In a separate bowl, mix buffalo sauce and melted butter.

6. Toss in Buffalo Sauce:
   - Once baked, transfer the cauliflower to a large bowl, pour the buffalo sauce mixture over the florets, and toss until evenly coated.

7. Serve:
   - Transfer the Buffalo Cauliflower Bites to a serving plate. Garnish with fresh parsley if desired. Serve with ranch or blue cheese dressing for dipping.

 Nutritional Information (per serving):

- Calories: 220 kcal
- Protein: 5g
- Fat: 7g
- Carbohydrates: 36g
- Fiber: 4g

Note: Nutritional information is approximate and may vary based on specific ingredients used.

Almond Butter and Celery Sticks

Prep Time: 5 minutes
Total Time: 5 minutes
Servings: 2

Ingredients:

- 4 celery stalks, cleaned and cut into sticks
- 1/2 cup almond butter
- Optional toppings: Chia seeds, sliced strawberries, or a drizzle of honey

Instructions:

1. Prepare Celery Sticks:
   - Clean the celery stalks and cut them into sticks of your preferred size.

2. Serve with Almond Butter:
   - Spread almond butter onto each celery stick.

3. Optional Toppings:
   - If desired, sprinkle chia seeds on top for added crunch, or add sliced strawberries for a fruity twist. For a touch of sweetness, drizzle honey over the sticks.

4. Serve:
   - Arrange the almond butter-filled celery sticks on a serving plate and enjoy!

Nutritional Information (per serving):

- Calories: 250 kcal
- Protein: 8g
- Fat: 21g
- Carbohydrates: 10g
- Fiber: 6g

Note: Nutritional information is approximate and may vary based on specific ingredients used.

Smoked Salmon Cucumber Rounds

Prep Time: 15 minutes
Total Time: 15 minutes
Servings: 4

Ingredients:

- 1 English cucumber, thinly sliced into rounds
- 4 oz smoked salmon
- 1/4 cup cream cheese, softened
- 1 tablespoon fresh dill, chopped
- 1 teaspoon capers
- Lemon zest for garnish
- Fresh chives for garnish (optional)

Instructions:

1. Prepare Cucumber Rounds:
   - Slice the English cucumber into thin rounds.

2. Assemble Smoked Salmon:
   - Place a small amount of softened cream cheese on each cucumber round.

3. Add Smoked Salmon:
   - Top the cream cheese with a piece of smoked salmon.

4. Garnish:
   - Sprinkle chopped fresh dill over the smoked salmon. Add a few capers on top.

5. Zest of Lemon:
   - Grate lemon zest over the rounds for a burst of citrus flavor.

6. Optional Chives:
   - Garnish with fresh chives if desired.

7. Serve:
   - Arrange the Smoked Salmon Cucumber Rounds on a serving platter and serve immediately.

Nutritional Information (per serving):

- Calories: 120 kcal
- Protein: 8g
- Fat: 9g
- Carbohydrates: 2g
- Fiber: 1g

Note: Nutritional information is approximate and may vary based on specific ingredients used.

Greek Yogurt with Berries and Nuts

Prep Time: 5 minutes
Total Time: 5 minutes
Servings: 2

Ingredients:
- 1 cup Greek yogurt
- 1 cup mixed berries (such as blueberries, strawberries, raspberries)
- 2 tablespoons chopped nuts (almonds, walnuts, or pecans)
- 1 tablespoon honey or maple syrup (optional)
- Fresh mint leaves for garnish (optional)

Instructions:
1. Prepare Greek Yogurt:
   - Spoon Greek yogurt into serving bowls.

2. Add Mixed Berries:
   - Arrange a generous portion of mixed berries on top of the Greek yogurt.

3. Sprinkle Chopped Nuts:
   - Sprinkle chopped nuts (almonds, walnuts, or pecans) over the berries.

4. Optional Sweetener:
   - If desired, drizzle honey or maple syrup over the yogurt and berries for added sweetness.

5. Garnish with Mint:

- Garnish with fresh mint leaves for a burst of freshness.

6. Serve:
   - Serve the Greek Yogurt with Berries and Nuts immediately and enjoy!

 Nutritional Information (per serving):
- Calories: 250 kcal
- Protein: 15g
- Fat: 10g
- Carbohydrates: 30g
- Fiber: 5g
Note: Nutritional information is approximate and may vary based on specific ingredients used.

Desserts

Chocolate Avocado Mousse

Prep Time: 10 minutes
Chill Time: 2 hours
Total Time: 2 hours 10 minutes
Servings: 4

Ingredients:

- 2 ripe avocados, peeled and pitted
- 1/4 cup cocoa powder
- 1/4 cup almond milk (or any milk of your choice)
- 1/4 cup maple syrup or agave nectar
- 1 teaspoon vanilla extract
- Pinch of salt
- Optional toppings: Whipped cream, berries, or shaved chocolate

Instructions:

1. Blend Avocados:
   - In a blender or food processor, combine the ripe avocados, cocoa powder, almond milk, maple syrup (or agave nectar), vanilla extract, and a pinch of salt.

2. Blend Until Smooth:
   - Blend the ingredients until smooth and creamy, scraping down the sides as needed.

3. Chill:
   - Transfer the chocolate avocado mixture to serving glasses or bowls. Cover and refrigerate for at least 2 hours to allow the mousse to chill and firm up.

4. Serve:
   - Once chilled, remove from the refrigerator and serve the Chocolate Avocado Mousse with your choice of toppings, such as whipped cream, berries, or shaved chocolate.

Nutritional Information (per serving):

- Calories: 200 kcal
- Protein: 3g
- Fat: 14g
- Carbohydrates: 21g
- Fiber: 7g

Note: Nutritional information is approximate and may vary based on specific ingredients used.

Keto Cheesecake Bites

Prep Time: 15 minutes
Chill Time: 2 hours
Total Time: 2 hours 15 minutes
Servings: 12

Ingredients:

For the Crust:

- 1 cup almond flour
- 3 tablespoons melted butter
- 1 tablespoon powdered erythritol (or your preferred keto-friendly sweetener)
- 1/2 teaspoon vanilla extract

For the Cheesecake Filling:

- 8 oz cream cheese, softened
- 1/3 cup powdered erythritol
- 1 teaspoon vanilla extract
- 1 large egg, room temperature

Optional Topping:

- Sugar-free fruit preserves or fresh berries

Instructions:

For the Crust:

1. Preheat Oven:
   - Preheat the oven to 325°F (163°C). Line a mini muffin tin with paper liners.

2. Mix **Ingredients:**
   - In a bowl, combine almond flour, melted butter, powdered erythritol, and vanilla extract. Mix until well combined.

3. Form Crust:
   - Spoon about 1 tablespoon of the mixture into each mini muffin cup. Press the mixture down to form a crust.

4. Bake:
   - Bake the crusts in the preheated oven for 8-10 minutes or until they are just starting to turn golden. Remove from the oven and let them cool.

For the Cheesecake Filling:

1. Prepare Filling:
   - In a separate bowl, beat together softened cream cheese, powdered erythritol, vanilla extract, and the egg until smooth.

2. Fill Muffin Cups:
   - Spoon the cream cheese mixture over the cooled crusts in the mini muffin tin.

3. Bake Again:
   - Bake in the oven for 15-18 minutes or until the cheesecake filling is set.

4. Chill:
   - Allow the cheesecake bites to cool in the tin, then transfer them to the refrigerator to chill for at least 2 hours.

5. Serve:
   - Once chilled, remove the Keto Cheesecake Bites from the refrigerator. Optionally, top each bite with a small dollop of sugar-free fruit preserves or fresh berries.

Nutritional Information (per serving):

- Calories: 150 kcal
- Protein: 4g
- Fat: 14g
- Carbohydrates: 3g
- Fiber: 1g

Note: Nutritional information is approximate and may vary based on specific ingredients used.

Coconut Almond Energy Balls

Prep Time: 15 minutes
Chill Time: 30 minutes
Total Time: 45 minutes
Servings: 12

Ingredients:

- 1 cup almonds, raw
- 1 cup shredded coconut, unsweetened
- 1/4 cup almond butter
- 1/4 cup coconut oil, melted
- 2 tablespoons chia seeds
- 1 teaspoon vanilla extract
- Pinch of salt

Instructions:

1. Prepare Almonds:
   - In a food processor, pulse the raw almonds until finely ground.

2. Combine Ingredients:
   - Add shredded coconut, almond butter, melted coconut oil, chia seeds, vanilla extract, and a pinch of salt to the ground almonds in the food processor.

3. Blend:
   - Pulse the mixture until well combined and forms a sticky dough.

4. Form Balls:
   - Scoop out tablespoon-sized portions of the mixture and roll them into compact balls using your hands.

5. Chill:
   - Place the coconut almond energy balls on a tray lined with parchment paper and refrigerate for at least 30 minutes to firm up.

6. Serve:
   - Once chilled, the energy balls are ready to be enjoyed. Store any leftovers in an airtight container in the refrigerator.

 Nutritional Information (per serving):

- Calories: 150 kcal
- Protein: 4g
- Fat: 14g
- Carbohydrates: 5g
- Fiber: 3g

Note: Nutritional information is approximate and may vary based on specific ingredients used.

Berries and Cream Parfait

Prep Time: 15 minutes
Total Time: 15 minutes
Servings: 2

Ingredients:

For the Vanilla Yogurt Layer:

- 1 cup Greek yogurt
- 1 tablespoon honey or maple syrup
- 1 teaspoon vanilla extract

For the Berry Layer:

- 1 cup mixed berries (strawberries, blueberries, raspberries)
- 1 tablespoon honey or maple syrup

For the Whipped Cream:

- 1/2 cup heavy cream
- 1 tablespoon powdered sugar (optional)
- 1/2 teaspoon vanilla extract

For Garnish:

- Fresh mint leaves (optional)

Instructions:

Vanilla Yogurt Layer:

1. Mix Ingredients:
    - In a bowl, combine Greek yogurt, honey or maple syrup, and vanilla extract. Mix well.

2. Assemble Parfait:
    - Spoon a layer of the vanilla yogurt into the bottom of serving glasses or bowls.

Berry Layer:

1. Sweeten Berries:
    - In another bowl, mix the mixed berries with honey or maple syrup.

2. Add Berry Layer:
    - Spoon a layer of the sweetened mixed berries on top of the vanilla yogurt layer.

Whipped Cream:

1. Whip Cream:
    - In a separate bowl, whip the heavy cream until soft peaks form. If desired, add powdered sugar and vanilla extract during the whipping process.

2. Top with Whipped Cream:
    - Dollop the whipped cream on top of the berries.

Garnish:

1. Optional Mint Leaves:

- Garnish with fresh mint leaves if desired.

2. Serve:
   - Serve the Berries and Cream Parfait immediately and enjoy!

 Nutritional Information (per serving):

- Calories: 300 kcal
- Protein: 10g
- Fat: 18g
- Carbohydrates: 30g
- Fiber: 4g

Note: Nutritional information is approximate and may vary based on specific ingredients used.

Sugar-Free Chocolate Bark with Nuts

Prep Time: 15 minutes
Chill Time: 1 hour
Total Time: 1 hour 15 minutes
Servings: 8

Ingredients:

- 1 cup sugar-free dark chocolate chips or chopped sugar-free dark chocolate
- 1/2 cup mixed nuts (almonds, walnuts, pecans), chopped
- 1/4 cup unsweetened shredded coconut
- 1/4 cup sugar-free dried cranberries or other sugar-free dried berries
- 1/2 teaspoon vanilla extract
- Pinch of sea salt

Instructions:

1. Prepare Baking Sheet:
   - Line a baking sheet with parchment paper.

2. Melt Chocolate:
   - In a heatproof bowl, melt the sugar-free dark chocolate using a double boiler or microwave in 30-second intervals, stirring until smooth.

3. Add Vanilla Extract:
   - Stir in the vanilla extract into the melted chocolate.

4. Spread Chocolate on Sheet:
   - Pour the melted chocolate onto the prepared baking sheet and spread it into an even layer.

5. Add Toppings:
   - Sprinkle the chopped nuts, shredded coconut, and sugar-free dried cranberries over the melted chocolate. Lightly press the toppings into the chocolate.

6. Chill:
   - Place the baking sheet in the refrigerator and chill for at least 1 hour or until the chocolate is completely set.

7. Break into Pieces:
   - Once set, break the sugar-free chocolate bark into pieces using your hands or a knife.

8. Serve:
   - Serve the Sugar-Free Chocolate Bark with Nuts immediately or store in an airtight container in the refrigerator.

Nutritional Information (per serving):

- Calories: 120 kcal
- Protein: 2g
- Fat: 10g
- Carbohydrates: 8g
- Fiber: 3g

Note: Nutritional information is approximate and may vary based on specific ingredients used.

Peanut Butter Chocolate Fat Bombs

Prep Time: 15 minutes
Chill Time: 2 hours
Total Time: 2 hours 15 minutes
Servings: 12

Ingredients:

For the Peanut Butter Layer:

- 1/2 cup natural peanut butter
- 1/4 cup coconut oil, melted
- 2 tablespoons powdered erythritol (or your preferred keto-friendly sweetener)
- 1/2 teaspoon vanilla extract
- Pinch of salt

For the Chocolate Layer:

- 1/2 cup sugar-free dark chocolate chips or chopped sugar-free dark chocolate
- 2 tablespoons coconut oil

Instructions:

Peanut Butter Layer:

1. Mix **Ingredients:**
   - In a bowl, mix together natural peanut butter, melted coconut oil, powdered erythritol, vanilla extract, and a pinch of salt until well combined.

2. Fill Molds:
   - Spoon the peanut butter mixture into silicone molds, filling each mold halfway. Smooth the top with a spatula.

3. Chill:
   - Place the molds in the freezer for about 30 minutes to firm up the peanut butter layer.

Chocolate Layer:

1. Melt Chocolate:
   - In a heatproof bowl, melt the sugar-free dark chocolate chips or chopped chocolate along with coconut oil. Stir until smooth.

2. Top with Chocolate:
   - Remove the molds from the freezer and spoon the melted chocolate over the peanut butter layer, covering it completely.

3. Chill Again:
   - Place the molds back in the freezer for at least 1-2 hours, or until the fat bombs are completely set.

4. Serve:
   - Once set, pop the Peanut Butter Chocolate Fat Bombs out of the molds and serve. Store any leftovers in the refrigerator.

Nutritional Information (per serving):

- Calories: 150 kcal
- Protein: 3g
- Fat: 14g
- Carbohydrates: 5g
- Fiber: 3g

Note: Nutritional information is approximate and may vary based on specific ingredients used.

Chia Seed Pudding with Vanilla and Almond Milk

Prep Time: 5 minutes
Chill Time: 4 hours or overnight
Total Time: 4 hours 5 minutes
Servings: 2

Ingredients:

- 1/4 cup chia seeds
- 1 cup unsweetened almond milk
- 1 tablespoon maple syrup or sweetener of choice
- 1/2 teaspoon vanilla extract
- Sliced almonds and fresh berries for topping (optional)

Instructions:

1. Mix Ingredients:
   - In a bowl, combine chia seeds, unsweetened almond milk, maple syrup, and vanilla extract. Stir well to ensure the chia seeds are evenly distributed.

2. Chill:
   - Cover the bowl and refrigerate for at least 4 hours or preferably overnight. This allows the chia seeds to absorb the liquid and create a pudding-like consistency.

3. Stir Before Serving:

- Before serving, give the chia pudding a good stir to break up any clumps and achieve a smooth texture.

4. Top with Almonds and Berries:
   - If desired, top the chia seed pudding with sliced almonds and fresh berries for added texture and flavor.

5. Serve:
   - Spoon the Chia Seed Pudding with Vanilla and Almond Milk into serving bowls and enjoy!

Nutritional Information (per serving):

- Calories: 120 kcal
- Protein: 3g
- Fat: 7g
- Carbohydrates: 12g
- Fiber: 7g

Note: Nutritional information is approximate and may vary based on specific ingredients used.

Avocado Chocolate Pudding

Prep Time: 10 minutes
Chill Time: 1 hour
Total Time: 1 hour 10 minutes
Servings: 4

Ingredients:

- 2 ripe avocados
- 1/4 cup unsweetened cocoa powder
- 1/4 cup almond milk (or any milk of choice)
- 1/4 cup maple syrup or sweetener of choice
- 1 teaspoon vanilla extract
- Pinch of salt
- Fresh berries or sliced fruits for garnish (optional)

Instructions:

1. Prepare Avocados:
   - Cut the ripe avocados in half, remove the pits, and scoop the flesh into a blender or food processor.

2. Add **Ingredients:**
   - Add cocoa powder, almond milk, maple syrup, vanilla extract, and a pinch of salt to the blender or food processor.

3. Blend Until Smooth:
   - Blend the ingredients until smooth and creamy. Scrape down the sides as needed to ensure everything is well incorporated.

4. Chill:
   - Transfer the avocado chocolate mixture into serving bowls or glasses. Cover and refrigerate for at least 1 hour to allow the pudding to set.

5. Garnish and Serve:
   - Before serving, garnish the Avocado Chocolate Pudding with fresh berries or sliced fruits if desired.

6. Enjoy:
   - Serve and enjoy this rich and indulgent chocolate pudding made with the goodness of avocados!

Nutritional Information (per serving):

- Calories: 220 kcal
- Protein: 3g
- Fat: 15g
- Carbohydrates: 25g
- Fiber: 7g

Note: Nutritional information is approximate and may vary based on specific ingredients used.

Lemon Coconut Bliss Balls

Prep Time: 15 minutes
Chill Time: 1 hour
Total Time: 1 hour 15 minutes
Servings: 12

Ingredients:

- 1 cup shredded coconut (plus extra for coating)
- 1 cup almond meal
- Zest of 1 lemon
- 3 tablespoons lemon juice
- 3 tablespoons coconut oil, melted
- 2 tablespoons maple syrup or sweetener of choice
- 1 teaspoon vanilla extract
- Pinch of salt

Instructions:
1. Combine Dry Ingredients:
   - In a bowl, combine shredded coconut, almond meal, and a pinch of salt.

2. Add Wet Ingredients:
   - Add lemon zest, lemon juice, melted coconut oil, maple syrup, and vanilla extract to the dry ingredients.

3. Mix Thoroughly:
   - Mix the ingredients thoroughly until well combined. The mixture should be sticky and easily moldable.

4. Shape into Balls:
   - Take small portions of the mixture and roll them
into balls between your palms. Adjust the size based
on your preference.

5. Coat with Coconut:
      - Roll the bliss balls in additional shredded
coconut to coat them evenly.

6. Chill:
      - Place the Lemon Coconut Bliss Balls in the
refrigerator for at least 1 hour to allow them to firm
up.

7. Serve:
      - Once chilled, serve and enjoy these zesty and
coconut-infused bliss balls!

 Nutritional Information (per serving):

- Calories: 120 kcal
- Protein: 2g
- Fat: 10g
- Carbohydrates: 6g
- Fiber: 2g

Note: Nutritional information is approximate and
may vary based on specific ingredients used.

Strawberry Almond Flour Mug Cake

Prep Time: 5 minutes
Cook Time: 2 minutes
Total Time: 7 minutes
Servings: 1

Ingredients:

- 3 tablespoons almond flour
- 1 tablespoon coconut flour
- 1/4 teaspoon baking powder
- Pinch of salt
- 2 tablespoons melted coconut oil
- 2 tablespoons unsweetened almond milk
- 1 tablespoon maple syrup or sweetener of choice
- 1/4 teaspoon vanilla extract
- 2-3 ripe strawberries, diced (plus extra for topping)

Instructions:

1. Prepare Mug:
   - Grease a microwave-safe mug with a bit of coconut oil.

2. Mix Dry Ingredients:
   - In a small bowl, whisk together almond flour, coconut flour, baking powder, and a pinch of salt.

3. Combine Wet Ingredients:

- In the mug, mix melted coconut oil, almond milk, maple syrup, and vanilla extract.

4. Add Dry Ingredients:
   - Gradually add the dry ingredients to the mug, stirring well to avoid lumps.

5. Add Diced Strawberries:
   - Gently fold in the diced strawberries into the batter.

6. Microwave:
   - Microwave the mug on high for 2 minutes or until the cake is set in the middle.

7. Top with Strawberries:
   - Allow the mug cake to cool for a minute before topping it with extra diced strawberries.

8. Serve:
   - Enjoy your Strawberry Almond Flour Mug Cake straight from the mug!

Nutritional Information (per serving):

- Calories: 350 kcal
- Protein: 5g
- Fat: 29g
- Carbohydrates: 18g
- Fiber: 5g

Note: Nutritional information is approximate and may vary based on specific ingredients used.

Smoothies

Green Keto Smoothie

Prep Time: 5 minutes
Total Time: 5 minutes
Servings: 1

Ingredients:

- 1 cup unsweetened almond milk
- 1/2 avocado, peeled and pitted
- 1 cup fresh spinach
- 1/2 cucumber, peeled and sliced
- 1/2 lemon, juiced
- 1 tablespoon chia seeds
- 1 tablespoon almond butter
- Ice cubes (optional)
- Sweetener of choice (optional)

Instructions:

1. Combine Ingredients:
   - In a blender, combine unsweetened almond milk, avocado, fresh spinach, cucumber, lemon juice, chia seeds, and almond butter.

2. Blend Until Smooth:
   - Blend the ingredients until smooth and creamy. If the smoothie is too thick, you can add more almond milk to reach your desired consistency.

3. Add Ice Cubes (Optional):
   - If you prefer a colder smoothie, add ice cubes to the blender and blend until the ice is crushed and the smoothie is well-chilled.

4. Sweeten to Taste (Optional):
   - Taste the smoothie and, if needed, add a keto-friendly sweetener of your choice to achieve the desired level of sweetness.

5. Serve:
   - Pour the Green Keto Smoothie into a glass and serve immediately.

Nutritional Information (per serving):

- Calories: 300 kcal
- Protein: 7g
- Fat: 25g
- Carbohydrates: 15g
- Fiber: 9g

Note: Nutritional information is approximate and may vary based on specific ingredients used.

Berry Protein Blast

Prep Time: 5 minutes
Total Time: 5 minutes
Servings: 1

Ingredients:
- 1 cup unsweetened almond milk
- 1/2 cup mixed berries (strawberries, blueberries, raspberries)
- 1/2 cup plain Greek yogurt
- 1 scoop vanilla protein powder
- 1 tablespoon chia seeds
- 1 tablespoon almond butter
- Ice cubes (optional)
- Sweetener of choice (optional)

Instructions:
1. Combine Ingredients:
    - In a blender, combine unsweetened almond milk, mixed berries, plain Greek yogurt, vanilla protein powder, chia seeds, and almond butter.

2. Blend Until Smooth:
   - Blend the ingredients until smooth and creamy. If you prefer a colder smoothie, you can add ice cubes to the blender and blend until the ice is crushed.

3. Sweeten to Taste (Optional):

   - Taste the smoothie and, if needed, add a sweetener of your choice to achieve the desired level of sweetness.

4. Serve:
   - Pour the Berry Protein Blast into a glass and serve immediately.

 Nutritional Information (per serving):
- Calories: 350 kcal
- Protein: 30g
- Fat: 15g
- Carbohydrates: 25g
- Fiber: 8g
Note: Nutritional information is approximate and may vary based on specific ingredients used.

Chocolate Almond Butter Delight

Prep Time: 5 minutes
Total Time: 5 minutes
Servings: 1

Ingredients:

- 1 cup unsweetened almond milk
- 2 tablespoons almond butter
- 1 scoop chocolate protein powder
- 1 tablespoon unsweetened cocoa powder
- 1/2 teaspoon vanilla extract
- Ice cubes (optional)
- Sweetener of choice (optional)

Instructions:

1. Combine Ingredients:
    - In a blender, combine unsweetened almond milk, almond butter, chocolate protein powder, unsweetened cocoa powder, and vanilla extract.

2. Blend Until Smooth:
    - Blend the ingredients until smooth and well combined. If you prefer a colder drink, you can add ice cubes to the blender and blend until the ice is crushed.

3. Sweeten to Taste (Optional):

- Taste the mixture and, if needed, add a sweetener of your choice to achieve the desired level of sweetness.

4. Serve:
   - Pour the Chocolate Almond Butter Delight into a glass and serve immediately.

 Nutritional Information (per serving):

- Calories: 350 kcal
- Protein: 25g
- Fat: 20g
- Carbohydrates: 15g
- Fiber: 6g

Note: Nutritional information is approximate and may vary based on specific ingredients used.

Avocado Mint Chip Smoothie

Prep Time: 5 minutes
Total Time: 5 minutes
Servings: 1

Ingredients:

- 1 cup unsweetened almond milk
- 1/2 avocado, peeled and pitted
- 1/4 cup fresh mint leaves
- 1 scoop chocolate protein powder
- 1 tablespoon unsweetened cocoa powder
- 1/2 teaspoon peppermint extract
- Ice cubes (optional)
- Sweetener of choice (optional)
- Dark chocolate chips for garnish (optional)

Instructions:

1. Combine Ingredients:
   - In a blender, combine unsweetened almond milk, avocado, fresh mint leaves, chocolate protein powder, unsweetened cocoa powder, and peppermint extract.

2. Blend Until Smooth:
   - Blend the ingredients until smooth and well combined. If you prefer a colder smoothie, you can add ice cubes to the blender and blend until the ice is crushed.

3. Sweeten to Taste (Optional):
   - Taste the smoothie and, if needed, add a sweetener of your choice to achieve the desired level of sweetness.

4. Garnish (Optional):
   - Pour the smoothie into a glass and, if desired, garnish with a sprinkle of dark chocolate chips for a mint chip twist.

5. Serve:
   - Serve the Avocado Mint Chip Smoothie immediately and enjoy!

 Nutritional Information (per serving):

- Calories: 300 kcal
- Protein: 20g
- Fat: 18g
- Carbohydrates: 15g
- Fiber: 7g

Note: Nutritional information is approximate and may vary based on specific ingredients used.

Cinnamon Vanilla Protein Shake

Prep Time: 5 minutes
Total Time: 5 minutes
Servings: 1

Ingredients:
- 1 cup unsweetened almond milk
- 1 scoop vanilla protein powder
- 1/2 teaspoon ground cinnamon
- 1/2 teaspoon vanilla extract
- 1 tablespoon almond butter
- Ice cubes (optional)
- Sweetener of choice (optional)

Instructions:
1. Combine **Ingredients:**
    - In a blender, combine unsweetened almond milk, vanilla protein powder, ground cinnamon, vanilla extract, and almond butter.

2. Blend Until Smooth:
    - Blend the ingredients until smooth and well combined. If you prefer a colder shake, you can add ice cubes to the blender and blend until the ice is crushed.

3. Sweeten to Taste (Optional):
    - Taste the shake and, if needed, add a sweetener of your choice to achieve the desired level of sweetness.

4. Serve:
   - Pour the Cinnamon Vanilla Protein Shake into a glass and serve immediately.

 Nutritional Information (per serving):

- Calories: 250 kcal
- Protein: 25g
- Fat: 10g
- Carbohydrates: 15g
- Fiber: 3g
Note: Nutritional information is approximate and may vary based on specific ingredients used.

Strawberry Coconut Cream

Prep Time: 5 minutes
Total Time: 5 minutes
Servings: 1

Ingredients:
- 1 cup coconut milk (unsweetened)
- 1 cup fresh strawberries, hulled
- 1/2 cup coconut cream
- 1 tablespoon chia seeds
- 1/2 teaspoon vanilla extract
- Ice cubes (optional)
- Sweetener of choice (optional)

Instructions:
1. Combine Ingredients:
    - In a blender, combine coconut milk, fresh strawberries, coconut cream, chia seeds, and vanilla extract.

2. Blend Until Smooth:
    - Blend the ingredients until smooth and well combined. If you prefer a colder smoothie, you can add ice cubes to the blender and blend until the ice is crushed.

3. Sweeten to Taste (Optional):
    - Taste the smoothie and, if needed, add a sweetener of your choice to achieve the desired level of sweetness.

4. Serve:
   - Pour the Strawberry Coconut Cream Smoothie into a glass and serve immediately.

 Nutritional Information (per serving):

- Calories: 300 kcal
- Protein: 5g
- Fat: 25g
- Carbohydrates: 15g
- Fiber: 7g
Note: Nutritional information is approximate and may vary based on specific ingredients used.

Coffee and Almond Smoothie

Prep Time: 5 minutes
Total Time: 5 minutes
Servings: 1

Ingredients:

- 1 cup brewed coffee, cooled
- 1/2 cup unsweetened almond milk
- 1 scoop vanilla protein powder
- 1 tablespoon almond butter
- 1/2 teaspoon ground cinnamon
- Ice cubes (optional)
- Sweetener of choice (optional)

Instructions:

1. Brew Coffee:
   - Brew a cup of coffee and allow it to cool to room temperature or refrigerate for a quick chill.

2. Combine Ingredients:
   - In a blender, combine cooled brewed coffee, unsweetened almond milk, vanilla protein powder, almond butter, and ground cinnamon.

3. Blend Until Smooth:
   - Blend the ingredients until smooth and well combined. If you prefer a colder smoothie, you can add ice cubes to the blender and blend until the ice is crushed.

4. Sweeten to Taste (Optional):
    - Taste the smoothie and, if needed, add a sweetener of your choice to achieve the desired level of sweetness.

5. Serve:
    - Pour the Coffee and Almond Smoothie into a glass and serve immediately.

Nutritional Information (per serving):

- Calories: 250 kcal
- Protein: 20g
- Fat: 15g
- Carbohydrates: 10g
- Fiber: 3g

Note: Nutritional information is approximate and may vary based on specific ingredients used.

Blueberry Avocado Bliss

Prep Time: 5 minutes
Total Time: 5 minutes
Servings: 1

Ingredients:
- 1/2 cup blueberries (fresh or frozen)
- 1/2 avocado, peeled and pitted
- 1 cup unsweetened almond milk
- 1 scoop vanilla protein powder
- 1 tablespoon chia seeds
- 1/2 teaspoon honey or sweetener of choice (optional)
- Ice cubes (optional)

Instructions:
1. Combine Ingredients:
   - In a blender, combine blueberries, avocado, unsweetened almond milk, vanilla protein powder, and chia seeds.

2. Blend Until Smooth:
   - Blend the ingredients until smooth and well combined. If you prefer a colder smoothie, you can add ice cubes to the blender and blend until the ice is crushed.

3. Sweeten to Taste (Optional):
   - Taste the smoothie and, if desired, add honey or a sweetener of your choice to achieve the desired level of sweetness.

4. Serve:
   - Pour the Blueberry Avocado Bliss Smoothie into a glass and serve immediately.

 Nutritional Information (per serving):

- Calories: 300 kcal
- Protein: 20g
- Fat: 18g
- Carbohydrates: 20g
- Fiber: 10g
Note: Nutritional information is approximate and may vary based on specific ingredients used.

Raspberry Lemonade Refresher

Prep Time: 5 minutes
Total Time: 5 minutes
Servings: 1

Ingredients:

- 1 cup fresh or frozen raspberries
- Juice of 1 lemon
- 1 tablespoon honey or sweetener of choice
- 1 cup cold water
- Ice cubes
- Fresh mint leaves for garnish (optional)

Instructions:

1. Prepare Raspberry Lemonade Base:
   - In a blender, combine raspberries, lemon juice, honey, and cold water.

2. Blend Until Smooth:
   - Blend the ingredients until the mixture is smooth and well combined.

3. Strain (Optional):
   - If you prefer a smoother texture, you can strain the raspberry lemonade to remove the seeds.

4. Sweeten to Taste:

- Taste the raspberry lemonade and, if needed, add more honey or sweetener to achieve your preferred level of sweetness.

5. Serve Over Ice:
   - Pour the Raspberry Lemonade Refresher over ice cubes in a glass.

6. Garnish (Optional):
   - Garnish with fresh mint leaves for a burst of freshness.

7. Stir and Enjoy:
   - Stir the raspberry lemonade, and enjoy the refreshing and tangy flavors!

 Nutritional Information (per serving):

- Calories: 80 kcal
- Protein: 1g
- Fat: 0g
- Carbohydrates: 20g
- Fiber: 5g

Note: Nutritional information is approximate and may vary based on specific ingredients used.

Pumpkin Spice Smoothie

Prep Time: 5 minutes
Total Time: 5 minutes
Servings: 1

Ingredients:

- 1/2 cup canned pumpkin puree
- 1 frozen banana
- 1 cup unsweetened almond milk
- 1 scoop vanilla protein powder
- 1/2 teaspoon pumpkin spice blend
- 1 tablespoon almond butter
- Ice cubes (optional)
- Sweetener of choice (optional)
- Whipped cream and a sprinkle of cinnamon for garnish (optional)

Instructions:

1. Combine Ingredients:
   - In a blender, combine canned pumpkin puree, frozen banana, unsweetened almond milk, vanilla protein powder, pumpkin spice blend, and almond butter.

2. Blend Until Smooth:
   - Blend the ingredients until smooth and well combined. If you prefer a colder smoothie, you can add ice cubes to the blender and blend until the ice is crushed.

3. Sweeten to Taste (Optional):
   - Taste the smoothie and, if needed, add a sweetener of your choice to achieve the desired level of sweetness.

4. Serve:
  - Pour the Pumpkin Spice Smoothie into a glass.

5. Garnish (Optional):
   - Optionally, top the smoothie with whipped cream and a sprinkle of cinnamon for a festive touch.

6. Stir and Enjoy:
  - Stir the Pumpkin Spice Smoothie and savor the warm and comforting flavors!

Nutritional Information (per serving):

- Calories: 300 kcal
- Protein: 20g
- Fat: 15g
- Carbohydrates: 25g
- Fiber: 8g

Note: Nutritional information is approximate and may vary based on specific ingredients used.

Conclusion

As we reach the culmination of our journey through "Atkins Diet for Beginners," it's evident that the Atkins approach goes beyond a mere diet—it's a lifestyle transformation. By exploring the synergy of nutrition, time, and weight loss, we've uncovered the power of low-calorie living and cultivated a lasting, healthy lifestyle.

This comprehensive guide has equipped you with the tools to balance nutrition, sustain weight loss, and infuse vitality into every moment. With 110 delicious recipes, this book ensures a flavorful and satisfying Atkins experience.

Remember, the Atkins journey is not just about shedding pounds; it's about fostering lasting wellness. By understanding the principles, philosophy, and benefits of the Atkins diet, you've laid the foundation for a healthier and more vibrant life.

As you embark on this transformative journey, embrace the variety of recipes from hearty breakfasts to savory dinners, delightful snacks, and indulgent desserts. Each recipe is a testament to the richness of flavor that can be enjoyed while still adhering to the Atkins principles.

In crafting this guide, my aim has been to empower you with the knowledge and recipes to make the Atkins lifestyle a seamless part of your daily routine. Whether you're a beginner or someone seeking to reinvigorate your commitment to a low-carb lifestyle, "Atkins Diet for Beginners" is your trusted companion.

May this book be the catalyst for positive change in your life. Here's to health, wellness, and the boundless possibilities that come with embracing the Atkins way of living. Cheers to your journey towards a healthier, happier you!

Ask for review

Dear Readers,

I hope you've enjoyed exploring the world of balanced nutrition, sustainable weight loss, and delicious recipes in "Atkins Diet for Beginners." Your feedback is invaluable to me, and I would be honored to hear about your experience with the book.

If you found the information helpful, inspiring, or if the recipes brought new flavors to your kitchen, please consider leaving a review. Your honest thoughts can guide and support other readers on their journey to a healthier lifestyle.

To leave a review, simply visit the platform where you purchased the book, and share your insights. Your feedback contributes to the community and helps us grow together.

Thank you for being part of this journey, and I look forward to hearing from you!

Warm regards,
Thelma J. Curtis

www.ingramcontent.com/pod-product-compliance
Lightning Source LLC
Chambersburg PA
CBHW070918260726
48661CB00003B/747